Praise for *The*

'There's something quietly wonder[...]
this book. Beneath the deceptive [...]
wisdom here that doesn't quite kn[...]
but sort of works its way into you, until it feels part of you....I
think this could be the new *A New Earth*.'

— James Wallman, author of *Time And
How To Spend It* and *Stuffocation*

'*The Book of Rest* is a beautifully written and masterful guidebook
that eloquently shows us how to recognize and embody lasting peace
and well-being and awaken to our essential wholeness amidst the
challenges of our everyday lives. James Reeves and Gabrielle Brown's
heartfelt gentleness and masterful wisdom shine through in the
teachings they reveal in this seminal work. Both profound and
practical *The Book of Rest* is a treasure and pleasure to read for all
who wish to embrace a clear path to embodying their full potential
as authentically alive human beings. A must-read!'

— Richard Miller, PhD. Founder, iRest Institute and developer
of iRest Yoga Nidra Meditation

'*The Book of Rest* invites you to experience how the state of true,
deep rest is always available, for anyone, at any time. Beautifully
written and very accessible. I love it.'

— Esther Ekhart, founder of EkhartYoga.com

*****

'I'm a 43-year-old MD of a large insolvency practice, I have 120
staff and earn enough. Like many people who are in the kind of
position I am in, I'm also very stressed. I developed what was a

possibly unhealthy relationship with self-help books some years ago: I was always trying to meditate and be mindful, but it was only with your book that I reached 'that place'. That place between the breath in meditation, that place that only you could try and describe, that wonderful, wonderful place. I can't believe the simplicity and beauty of the method.'

— Danny Morris, reader

'I'm someone who tends towards anxiety and is easily overwhelmed, mostly by my own inner dialogue. For years I've perfected the art of escaping – at times through sugar, at times through binge-scrolling online, and at times, ironically, through yoga. After years of struggling with uncomfortable feelings and sensations in my body, of being depleted by my own reactivity to the world around me and within me, and by trying with every ounce of myself to control everything and make everything perfect because then I would find peace, I can say that I've relaxed my effort more than ever. Things that used to deeply trigger me now don't. I want to congratulate both of you for this beautiful work. You speak so many truths in this book; you speak of how simple, albeit not easy, it is to unveil the peace and freedom we are all longing for.'

— Sarah Maar, reader

'You provide a really wonderful space for just being, and nurturing the self, which is so very needed after the pandemic has left us reeling emotionally and facing many challenges, internal and external. I am a psychotherapist by profession and I find the psychological depth to the practices you are offering really excellent. The invitation to welcome and to be curious about difficult feelings is so very helpful. It is helping me personally and enriching me professionally too.'

— Femke Molekamp, reader

James Reeves and Gabrielle Brown are founders of Restful Being, a yoga and meditation school focused on the extraordinary power of rest to help people uncover their innate sense of steady, spacious calm. James is a world-leading trainer in yoga nidra, a transformative state of deep rest. He has been teaching yoga and meditation since 2005, working globally, online and even on-site at the Oscars. Gabrielle is primarily a writer and editor with over two decades' experience in communications and publishing. She has been practising yoga since she was a teenager and qualified to teach in 2013.

Thank you

Thanks to everyone at HQ for their enthusiasm and excitement at putting our work out there, specifically our publisher Lisa Milton and editor Kate Fox, and to our copyeditor Laura Herring for her invaluable observations. This book would not be happening if Anna Hogarty at Madeleine Milburn hadn't envisioned the title and everything it stands for, and thanks also to Hayley Steed and Madeleine for their ongoing support and encouragement. Jessica Harvey, for casting her superlatively creative eye over the cover design.

James: To my father, for your desire to understand the deeper meaning of life, and my mother, for living it with discreet beauty. My brother, Simon, for his big heart, and his partner Wayne, for his quiet strength. To Jayson, Justin and all my friends who have provided laughter and lightness to balance introversion and intensity. To my beloved teacher, Richard Miller, for living these teachings with such grace and kindness, and the broader iRest community for your examples of how to be damn good human beings.

Gabrielle: Thanks to my mother, Marie-France, who introduced me not only to yoga but also to James. My father, Robin, who has always encouraged me to see how fundamental the written word is in understanding and augmenting our experience of being human. My siblings, Thomas, Scott and Sophie – my comrades in life. Filkins Book Club for over a decade of good company and making me read things I didn't think I wanted to read. To all my yoga and meditation teachers for helping me feel comfortable in body and mind, and to Beth, Jude, and Jess for always being there.

THE
BOOK
OF
REST

*How to find calm
in a chaotic world*

JAMES REEVES AND GABRIELLE BROWN

ONE PLACE. MANY STORIES

HQ
An imprint of HarperCollins*Publishers* Ltd
1 London Bridge Street
London SE1 9GF

This edition 2021

1
First published in Great Britain by
HQ, an imprint of HarperCollins*Publishers* Ltd 2019

ISBN: 978-0-00-832166-6

Printed and bound in Great Britain by CPI Group (UK) Ltd, Croydon CR0 4YY

MIX
Paper from
responsible sources
FSC **FSC™ C007454**
www.fsc.org

This book is produced from independently certified FSC™ paper
to ensure responsible forest management.

For more information visit: www.harpercollins.co.uk/green

Contents

For Poppy and Luca. You are perfect.

Introduction

We're going to take you on a journey to your most rested self.

We're going to show you that whatever you have going on in your life right now, part of you is always at rest. Part of you is completely calm, completely balanced, completely satisfied and completely shatterproof.

This is a journey that anyone can go on. You don't need to know anything. You don't need to do anything in preparation. You don't need any kit. You don't need any skills. You don't need a particular body, diet or mindset. You don't need any particular kind of anything to take this journey.

You only need you. Exactly as you are, right now, however you are.

You're already ready.

***

Whether you're sleep deprived, stressed, ill, agitated or even just grappling with a nagging feeling that something isn't quite right, you are still, deep within yourself, just as OK as absolutely everyone else alive right now. At the very depths of your being, there is no resistance, tension or tiredness. There is no judgement, pain or fear. This is the very essence of who you are.

But we know this might not be a possibility you can entertain right now.

At no point on this journey do you have to 'get your head' around anything or force yourself into taking on a particular attitude. This is a book of gentle enquiry and incidental experience. It should require little effort other than the act of reading itself.

On the surface of things, the subject of rest might appear to be about taking a nap or getting more sleep or perhaps even kicking back with a glass of wine, but while these are some of our most favourite things to do and can benefit us in many ways, they can also distract us from the true experience of rest.

In the same way, although we are teachers of yoga and meditation and practise them often, these techniques are not in themselves always restful or always peaceful. Methods like these are intended to help us find a sense of space within our lives, but for many people they instead end up becoming something else we are *adding* to our experience. They become loaded with more actions, goals, frustrations and desires. . . this is not restful.

Perhaps you've tried yoga or meditation or other practices that you thought would leave you feeling more rested; perhaps you haven't.

It doesn't matter. Our aim is not to train you in any of these but instead take you straight to the heart of the very thing they attempt to point towards: the constant unchanging awareness that lies at the heart of your existence.

We're going to demonstrate that rest, and being restful, is something that is always there within you, rather than something you must weave into your experience.

How can we show you how to do nothing?

Being able to recognise and allow true rest is vital to us feeling whole, authentic and balanced. When we stop, we are able to experience the stillness that exists between and beyond our thoughts and self-narrative. Very often, we catch only a glimpse of this stillness, but this is all we need to see to know that it is there and, ultimately, if you're willing to go all the way with us here, that it is who we really are.

Many self-help books provide the tools to go off and change your life. We hope you will read *this* book and, in the experience alone, see that the calm that you think will come when you've got it all worked out is already here. You're just too busy *trying* to see it, to see it.

We will constantly urge you to do nothing. We will repeatedly reassure you that you, the world and the people around you have everything to gain from you doing nothing.

— *Rest needs you to do nothing.*

You will have had many moments of 'doing nothing' in your life before now, but what's different is that you might not have turned your attention to this act of stopping before or how you felt during those moments. You might not even have noticed that you had stopped or thought about what that stopping *was*.

As we turn our attention to rest, we can explore what it's like, and we will likely discover (or uncover) a place where everything can be welcomed, without condition, judgement or objective. A place where we are *always* welcome. How often does that happen in life?

Rest might seem ungraspable, but it is always here

This restful quality we're pointing to is hard to pin down. The challenge is that it isn't a thing. It's no-thing. *Nothing*.

It's not something that you *do*; it's something that's always the case. You cannot get hold of it, you cannot *grasp* this restfulness because it's here right now, behind and around all your thoughts.

It's near impossible to imagine something that has no qualities. Something that by definition is necessarily indescribable. Therefore, our task now is to take you beyond your thoughts, beyond your imaginings, and into the experience of rest itself. Everything we present and any practices we have set out here are based on experience, very intentionally, to mirror this non-thing.

— *No-thing is best met by nothing.*

Being restful towards rest

In truth, rest is not something that can be guaranteed. You can be led to the door of rest, but nothing can open that door. The fact is, the door will open itself and, as long as you're allowing, you will fall into the stillness beyond. Some find it easy to access this 'quietness', while others find it harder to get past distractions. You might stumble upon it while a-top the number 7 bus and yet find it elusive when you formally set out to do nothing.

Falling into this feeling of stillness can happen to anybody, at any time, but there are gentle approaches that might make you more prone to fall, or to more easily stumble into it. Knowing and reconnecting with this deepest quality of who you are can be a happy accident, springing out of nowhere, but we hope it might also be helped along with the suggestions in this book.

Are some people better at resting than others?

Because rest is a matter of doing nothing, anyone can rest as long as they are willing to let go of the idea that they must 'do' something to make it happen, or that they must somehow *make* themselves more 'peaceful'. People who have been practising yoga, meditation or mindfulness for a number of years have not somehow banked any more 'inner peace' than Mrs Jones whose preferred relaxation technique is hitting the local bingo hall, they simply may know how to access it more readily. They are no more (or less) at peace at their core than you are, even as you read this and perhaps even believe that you've never been at rest in your life.

Those of us who actively engage in formal relaxation techniques (or whatever you want to call them) are simply those of us who sought out or discovered a particular process that helped us to stop, or that helped us to believe that all we had to do was stop. Once we experienced the benefits of stopping, and then falling into that stillness, we continued to stop and do nothing as often as life allowed.

A popular assumption that we regularly come across is that because we teach yoga we are inherently calm, whereas the opposite is just as (or perhaps more) likely to be true. Look at any yoga teacher's website and read through their bio and you'll typically see a story that begins with a person who, at a particularly low and stressful point in their lives, when all else failed, found yoga to be the only thing that helped bring them back to a place of physical and mental OK-ness. You rarely read a bio that speaks of a blissful childhood, harmonious adolescence, super-chilled career path and a sudden realisation of, 'I really ought to share my naturally easy-going demeanour with the world.'

We 'teachers of rest' were at one time likely to have been extremely rest*less* – perhaps even addicted to restlessness – and then, by various routes and accidental happenings, we discovered our innate restfulness.

You might find the techniques and processes in this book help lead you to the door of your innate stillness, or you might find you can feel your way towards it more instinctively. The rested self doesn't care how you find it. All practices are a path to rest, but they are not rest in themselves (and although there are many paths to rest, none of them is necessary to you feeling rested).

We are aware that we are in danger of shooting ourselves in the foot by declaring that you do not need to understand complicated yoga, meditation or mindfulness techniques to feel rested. Although we earn a living helping people to feel rested, much of our work is about helping shake off the idea that we must study, practise, understand, master or refine anything to find peace within ourselves. Ours is a business that can sometimes seem mysterious and indeed mystic – full of methods and teachings that only a few special gurus have mastered and are able to share. While we know that there are some beings out there with certainly unusual and perhaps even magical abilities, they do not somehow bestow upon their followers a more special kind of peace than you are capable of finding by other means – either with somebody's help, or by simply sitting alone by yourself.

We don't mean to pitch *The Wizard of Oz* as a life handbook, but the story's message is relevant to the above point. All the while Dorothy seeks a guru (the Wizard) to show her the way home, she already has everything she needs about her person to find the way home herself. Indeed, the Wizard is an illusion, or at least a human no different to Dorothy. However, that's not to say the Wizard didn't help Dorothy uncover this fact. She first had to see that her beliefs were nothing more than an illusion before she could tap (three times) into her own inner knowing.

Rest, yoga and yoga nidra

While yoga as a largely physical practice has now become an established part of our culture in the West, the 'rest' aspect of this ancient tradition, known as yoga nidra, has recently started to attract interest as a standalone practice. As much as we can assure you that you do not need to develop particular skills or have access to a guru to find rest, if there is one undertaking that might offer some kind of fast track to rest (in that it takes you by the hand and leads you, without you perhaps even realising it), then yoga nidra is our winning contender, and we have included a number of self-enquiry practices in this book that take inspiration from the yoga nidra techniques we share in our classes and training courses.

Like many yogis, our journey started with an interest in the physical aspect of the practice and all the tangible benefits it can bring, though in time we realised something far more interesting was unveiling itself. For most of us, a yoga practice means working through a series of asanas (postures), and we feel secure in the knowledge that we are 'doing' something and that we will therefore likely see results. Certainly we start to see physical changes, and this is pleasing, but because when we are working ourselves into the postures we use our breath to help sustain our position and, especially in postures that require balance, we find our minds quieten as we focus on remaining steady and still, we might also notice a subtle sense of calm reveals itself to us – one that perhaps stays with us even after our practice. However, many of us become distracted by the movement aspect of yoga and continue our 'yoga journey' by aiming to become stronger, spend longer in headstands, be able to touch the floor without bending our knees, etc. Although that glimpse of calm pops in and out of the practice and our life beyond, almost saying, 'Hey, I'm here! You don't need to spend five minutes upside down to see me!', we plough on, developing that back bend into something that looks quite spectacular and has everyone applauding our commitment to. . . to our backbend, perhaps.

A 'physical' yoga practice can lead you to the contrastingly still aspect of your experience, but this 'restful awareness' can equally be uncovered with very subtle explorations of the body and breath, and by enquiring into your feelings, emotions, thoughts and beliefs as a means to discover what lies *beyond* them. A class in which students are simply welcomed to allow whatever they are feeling – physical and emotional – to be present, just as it is, can be as 'enlightening' as several years of refining sequences of sophisticated physical postures.

Often referred to as 'sleep yoga' (though this isn't a particularly accurate term), yoga nidra is very much a process of surrendering. There is nothing to 'do' in a yoga nidra class other than be still and follow the teacher's words as they use various techniques to guide you into being somewhere between awake and asleep (if you've ever dozed on a beach, slipping in and out of waking-dreams all the while aware of the sound of seagulls and children playing around you then you'll know this state). We've had students describe yoga nidra as 'meditation by stealth', because by its very nature, you don't have to *do* anything and yet you find yourself doing something amazing.

For many, a yoga nidra class – or any 'not-doing class', for there is not necessarily any reason to label it – presents a terrifying prospect. The thought of lying down in a room for an hour with absolutely nothing required other than that you be present with yourself can be an incredibly uncomfortable proposition. You can't hide from yourself, you might have to listen to yourself and you might see aspects of yourself that you have perhaps been distracting yourself from with other practices or exercises. This doesn't sound restful, but you cannot rest without stopping, and when we first stop, we may initially be bombarded with inner noise, not inner peace. This is all part of the journey to rest.

We've had students who, when they first attended a rest-based class, expressed concern that it wouldn't be enough for them. Their worry was that the focus on effortlessness and lack of physical exertion meant there couldn't possibly be any benefits. But such classes offer many people a rare chance to welcome their inner noise, and be present with themselves in a way that is deeply transformative, leaving you feeling more rested and refreshed than we would argue any form of exercise could.

That said, regardless of our respect and love for the practice, we did not want this book to be a yoga nidra handbook, because we want you to know, and wish to prove to you, that you do not need anything – not even yoga nidra – to rest. Yoga nidra has certainly been a core vehicle in helping us uncover our already-rested nature, but we know we can throw it away and our rested nature will still be there. Practising yoga nidra might help you connect with your innate stillness, but that stillness already exists within you. That stillness is yours.

How to approach our self-enquiry practices

Rest is the most natural state of simply 'being'. It happens to us when we stop and it reminds us that there is more to us than our thinking, doing and feeling experiences – rest allows us to uncover our awareness. The self-enquiries in this book are intended to help you slip into your own awareness, without effort. For this reason, they should be approached with a degree of lightness. There is no right or wrong way to undertake them.

You can think of them as experiments, without any expected outcome. You will likely face challenges, such as meeting incessant chatter of your mind or a particularly eccentric or nagging self-narrative, and while we understand this might be disconcerting we will, throughout the course of this journey, illustrate how to 'do nothing' about such apparent obstacles to your rest. (We are aware there is a contradiction here, in that we are going to show you how to do something so that you can ultimately do nothing. . .)

The enquiries might be useful in helping you to understand rest in the context of your body, mind and that which lies beyond, but we want you to know these are experiments in showing you what you already have; they are not methods to be mastered or skills to be sharpened. They can be employed by anyone and there is no reason why their 'results' shouldn't be as profound as techniques practised by experienced yogi or meditators (or witches, wizards, Munchkins, etc.).

They are exercises in observation, but they might just enable you to allow rest to come when you start feeling that tension between *wanting* to make rest happen and knowing that the more you try to rest, the further away you are from actually resting (if you've ever grappled with insomnia then you will be familiar with this challenge). Ultimately, our advice is that as you set about an enquiry, you let everything unfold just as it wishes. This is your new mantra. . . to let go of immediately.

Our purpose in this book is to demonstrate, time and again, that you already know how to find rest. You just have to trust that it is there and that any apparent obstacles to you being able to connect with it are completely normal.

A busy mind does not mean you are less able to connect with your innate peace, a period of turmoil does not diminish its presence, and nor does a week of pasta and Chianti in Tuscany or a best-forgotten experience in Vegas (definitely not).

We will constantly remind you that it is not us nor anyone nor anything else that is able to apply rest into your experience of life. There is no magic to this, no superpowers required. Rest is not something that can be transferred from one person to another, or from anything onto you.

We know, though, that no amount of us telling you that the very essence of your being is always at peace, always OK and completely shatterproof will convince you of this fact. In order for you to believe us you will have to experience it for yourself.

In order to take this journey with us you have to be prepared to let go of the urge to make anything happen. You have to trust that you do not need to understand, work out or work through anything. *You* do not need to change, because you already are everything you will ever be: beneath everything, you are complete and uncon-ditionally contented.

— *To go on this journey with us you must be willing to do only one thing: nothing.*

Absolutely nothing.

And you must absolutely not try to rest.

Trying, is not resting. Resting is doing nothing. It is *being*.

So, let's try this. Let's stop, let everything go (including any attempt to let things go), and begin.

Enquiry 1:
What happens if you do nothing?

We all struggle to stop, and then we convince ourselves that 'stopping' is something we must learn to do — an art to master. Stopping is, however, more of an exercise in *un*-learning, of learning not to resist the happenings of our mind, body and everything in between that invariably unravels when we stop. A course in meditation does not so much allow you to develop any skills, more, it gives you the support framework you might need in order to be still and merely *be* with whatever happens to you when you stop trying to do anything.

However, when most people sit for meditation there's often a desire for some kind of technique, some 'tricks' to help you stop and feel OK about stopping. One of the most confounding and at the same time liberating 'activities' that we do on our retreats is ask attendees to sit for half an hour and do nothing. We are often explicit with this and assert that under no circumstances should there be any meditating. This often creates a lot of confusion, particularly for those who have an established meditation practice or other formal route into the experiences that can come from meditation. There is a degree of discomfort when we suggest not that their techniques don't have purpose or are in any way wrong, but that it is possible that doing nothing can be as 'effective' as doing something.

On a recent retreat, after one of these 'do nothing' sessions, a participant shared their experience with the group, bemoaning that they were too distracted to do nothing — they could hear noise outside, became aware of their response to that noise, and then preoccupied by the thoughts that came after that. At this point a re-orientation was necessary and we asked the group to consider the possibility that although our attention wanders from thoughts to sounds to feelings and sensations, perhaps it's not that we are *doing* any of this but more that it's just *happening*. Doing nothing doesn't mean nothing will happen.

— *That we are doing nothing doesn't mean we should expect stillness or silence or comfort.*

Doing nothing is an act of allowing; it is effortless, though perhaps not easy. That said, once we can grasp this concept – that we need not do anything – the experience is then very relaxing. (It's not that we're *trying* to relax, it just happens as a result of letting go of all control and reactivity to our experience.) Letting everything be just as it is involves layers of letting go, until you happen to be *letting everything be as it is*, including your distinct inability to let everything be as it is. . .

- *Prepare yourself to do nothing. You might want to turn off your phone, close your computer, shut the curtains, or do whatever it takes to reduce the likelihood of you being disturbed (or disturbing yourself)*

- *Make yourself comfortable, either sitting or lying down – whatever feels best for you. Make sure it is in a position that can remain comfortable for the entire time you'll be resting,* so if this means an 'easy' posture (relaxed in the armchair) then this is better than some kind of formal 'meditation' posture

– Now, in the same way that you've taken a physical posture in preparation for doing nothing, take a similar posture in your mind (however this may come to you)

– Stay with this posture. This means really *not doing anything*. Do not edit or control your experience in any way. Don't watch the breath or count or think about a special something or someone. If you're used to using a technique to help calm the mind or focus your thoughts, then we invite you to try giving it up and see what happens

– Drop your expectations and see if you can let go of any need for an outcome

– Notice how your mind will want to do so many other things and think so many thoughts. Just let that happen. You don't have to do a thing

– If you find this really hard, start with just a minute or two and then build up slowly. Most people report a noticeable shift in their experience around the 20-minute mark, and again at 30 minutes. The enquiry will likely feel restless and noisy on and off before then

– Don't worry if you can't reach the 20- or 30-minute mark. Build your tolerance for nothing slowly over time

- Whenever you feel it is time to end this enquiry, mentally or physically mark the moment however you wish (a little stretch, a deep breath)

- As you 'resurface', notice what your immediate thoughts are about the enquiry, and then remind yourself that whatever your experience, you cannot have done anything wrong

- Notice how this period of 'nothing' impacts the rest of your day. What does 'nothing' bring to your life?

What Is Rest?

Rest is a naturally occurring phenomenon. It is the thing that happens between, behind and around all our experience. It is the space that appears, however fleetingly, between all of the activities, all of the stuff and all of the thoughts, and while we might not think it has any value, it is the glue that binds everything together.

By stopping and doing nothing for a while you can recover the ability to recognise this spaciousness and begin to feel spacious about life again.

Throughout this book we will be exploring the 'you' that exists beyond your thinking mind – the you that is part of the space between everything else. We will look at how rest is both a means to experience this aspect of your existence and also the results of being reminded of it.

In this and the following chapters we will consider the relationship between our feelings, experiences, rest, restfulness and this concept of 'being' over 'doing' – being in the moment, being aware, being mindful, being human (all the beings).

Along the way, we will come across many apparent contradictions and paradoxes. . . and then they will dissolve. . . so long as you don't try to figure them out.

— *We will go round in circles, and we will see that this was all part of the journey.*

You've probably heard the expression, 'at one with everything' or 'at one with the universe'. It's a phrase that seeks to capture that feeling of there being nothing in our experience that we wish to change. In these moments, we feel held, connected, resolved, at ease, open. There is no sense of conflict or resistance.

But in these moments, we are not actually thinking, 'I am the universe and the universe is me', because, most likely, we are *not thinking at all.*

Crucially, these moments don't always come the minute you buy that car you've had your heart set on or get that promotion or resolve that conflict with your cousin. They often come out of nowhere.

Which means it is possible this feeling of being 'at one' (of everything being completely OK), exists regardless of what we think, do and have. It is possible that at the essence of all our experience, is a pervading sense of everything being just as it should be.

There are countless words and expressions that point towards the 'state' and the 'thing' that lies beyond the mind and beyond experience. You might use 'consciousness' or 'awareness'. You may have heard of 'nondualism' and the 'non-dual state' – simply meaning 'not divided' ('not two'). Or if you're used to a more 'new age' vibe then there's 'source', 'soul' or 'white light'. Perhaps you've even come across the police-drama-sounding 'witness state'? And when describing what it feels like to be in this state, we might use words such as 'peaceful', 'blissful', or describe a sense of pervading stillness or feeling of balance and harmony.

Whether we use any or all of these terms or we make up our own, we can never accurately describe any of it because it is necessarily elusive. The state is a no-state and the feeling of being in it is nothing but pure *being*.

In this book, our preference is for 'essence' or 'essential self', and when we talk about connecting with it, we like to say we are 'being', but all these descriptions are merely our way of pointing to something that you ultimately need to experience yourself in all its word-less, thought-less glory. It might not have a name, but it's right there, in front of your nose (well, actually, it's behind your nose, and in front of it, too, and it's none and both of those things, it's what's *aware* of your nose. . . etc.).

When we rest, when we do nothing, we give ourselves the chance to go beyond our mind and beyond our experience. Ultimately, in moments of not doing and of experiencing only our awareness, we are in a state of one-ness. We don't feel the separateness of our bodies, the conflicts of our emotions, the differences between ourselves and others.

It is a difficult concept to get our heads around, since our minds love to objectify, to have a 'thing' to cling on to. We're all very uncomfortable with not knowing. We want to make this thing that cannot be named a thing. Our head really doesn't like what this *thing* implies: that it cannot control our individual experience of life.

You might already have your own understanding of consciousness, and have your own words for it, and perhaps even a different system for thinking about it. If you are attached to how you already think about this quality we are exploring, perhaps you could consider letting go of your current beliefs, or at least hold them a little less tightly.

— *We are not any one thing.*

Rest and theory

There is a history to the teachings and the terminology we are sharing with you (and then asking you to unlearn), but more importantly there is a mystery. Some traditions of yoga consider consciousness as being personal or separate from life itself, while other teachings called this theory into question and after further exploration determined it to be a quality that seems all pervasive. The yogis' experiences of awareness brought the insight that it was utterly impersonal, though entirely inclusive; that what we are at our most essential is actually universal, all pervasive and utterly unified.

If you enjoy particle physics (and what's not to love?!) then you'll know that science is forever changing and shifting its theory on what, ultimately, we're all made from (and by 'we', we mean us, the planet, the solar system and beyond – everything ever). Some theories are moving closer towards determining that we are all one and the same thing, flashing in and out of existence, in a space that is bound neither by space nor time. This is interesting in relation to what we're trying to point you towards in this book, but it's still just theory.

We cannot write about rest without discussing its apparent coun-teragent, *energy*. In the traditions from which many of our teachings come there are certainly references to energy that do not marry with the scientific observations on the subject. Science defines energy not as a 'thing' but as a measurement of an object's capacity for doing work, whereas new age and esoteric communi-ties talk about energy as though it were a separate entity – a 'life force' or 'qi' – capable of moving through time and space and affecting objects as it does, perhaps charging them up 'positively', or healing them somehow.

Some people expect yoga and meditation to take them on a journey where they will eventually experience some kind of heavenly fanfare and this life force will reveal itself to them. Some people believe they have special powers that enable them to see such forces. We can entertain the idea that they possibly do (and possibly don't), but that doesn't help the vast majority of us who either don't believe in such energy or do but have never witnessed it. We like to work with observations and enquiries that anyone can do right now.

Therefore, with a nod to a tradition that's at least 3,000 years old and a thumbs up to the science that is excited by the fact that everything might be the same thing, even though we have no idea what that thing is, we have permission to lean into the vast mystery that resides beyond current knowledge and reason.

Rest and your feelings

The times in our life when we feel most rested are the times when we are not wishing to change any particular aspect of our experience. And herein lies the problem: the times we feel most rested are the times when we need rest the least. When we're overwhelmed by our experiences and our feelings, our desire to control them becomes stronger, and we rest less. We are rest-*less*.

During the course of our lives, we have had spells of feeling wonderful, awful, bored, depressed, extraordinary, anxious, weird, ill and, occasionally, something that we might call *normal*. We suspect you have had a similar journey, and perhaps like us, you couldn't always put your finger on why you felt one way or another.

Feelings can be like that: unpredictable, unexpected, uncontrollable, unfathomable – all the uns.

How many times have you said to yourself after something you were dreading, 'That wasn't so bad!'? Or have you ever found yourself moved to tears quite unexpectedly by a film or book (or even an advert)? And what about anger? Intense rage can fire up out of nowhere – stubbing your toe, a snappy comment from a colleague who hits the wrong button (a button you maybe didn't even know you had), a slow driver when you're already cutting it fine.

And then there's anxiety, the tenacious destroyer of all things restful, coming at the most unexpected of times and leaving in just the same way.

ASK YOURSELF

Can you recall a time when an intense emotion came up seemingly out of nowhere?

Once we recognise that feelings are flighty fellows, we can become open to the possibility that there is not much to be gained from trying to control them. We might start to see that it is our incessant desire to control how we feel and control the experiences that we think will lead to us experiencing particular feelings that exhausts us and, ironically, leaves us feeling the very thing we wish not to feel.

Once we realise that how, why and when we feel the things we feel is not something we have all that much control over, we might want to ask ourselves if there is much point in becoming overly attached to or afraid of any of our feelings or the experiences we think they relate to. Feelings will come and go, and we'll rarely know exactly why.

With all these unforeseen feelings playing out as they seemingly so wish, there is, perhaps surprisingly, an opportunity to consider ourselves a little less at their mercy. There is the chance here to step back and notice an inherent calm amidst this chaos. Whenever we experience a feeling, we also *notice* it. We are aware of it coming and going. We watch it. We observe it. We provide a space in which it can play out, and then leave. So what is this space? Who is this 'watcher', this 'awareness'? What is this awareness *feeling*?

Is it possible that the part of you that is watching your feelings is not actually *feeling* your feelings?

Amidst the hurly-burly, chaotic, exhausting playing out of your emotions, is it possible that there is part of you – the deepest, most essential aspect of your being – that is always there *just watching*? Is it possible that regardless of what it is watching, this aspect of your being is always OK? It is always *at peace*? It is always just. . . being?

Rest requires us to give up any ideas about control: controlling our experiences, controlling our feelings and controlling how we rest. Rest is fundamentally effortless and detached from experience. Rest is, therefore, a means to connect with this always-at-ease awareness that is the essence of your existence – perhaps just to glimpse, perhaps to loiter. Ultimately, rest both connects you with this ease and reminds you that it is there, that at your very depths, you are always restfully being.

Rest is what happens when everything else stops

We might at times want to call this state of watchful, restful, full-yet-empty being *peace* (even though it resides beyond peace. . .). We're not talking about a spiritual peace, or even a physical peace, but more a sense of absolute OK-ness – of absolute completeness – that very often comes out of nowhere and without us having done anything to prompt it. Sometimes, we don't realise it's been there until it's gone.

When this quality of peace becomes present in our experience it feels as though we have connected with something deep – something knowing – within ourselves, while at the same time we have a sense of being connected with everything we had thought was outside of ourselves. We, for just moments, become aware of our own smallness yet somehow feel greater for the realisation.

This quality of peace requires absolutely nothing for you to connect with it: and this is the problem. We very rarely do nothing. In fact, nothing is not something you can *do*.

That said, regardless of your circumstances, you will have experienced this quality of peace many times in your life already, however fleetingly, and without exception these will have all been times when you stopped trying to do anything (including trying to bring about a sense of peace). You will have been resting – that is, you will have separated yourself from the desire to do, have, think or feel anything at all.

Perhaps you woke up this morning and for those first few seconds were aware of a sense of ease and spaciousness before your brain kicked in and started barking orders at you or telling you stories about how you were going to feel for the remainder of the day. Or perhaps you recently undertook a task that consumed your full attention so much so that all your mind-chatter cleared out the way until it felt as if 'you', in effect, was gone. Perhaps you can recall having been to a music concert and suddenly feeling as though you and the musicians and the music were one; as though everyone in the venue had merged into the same poignant, unified experience. Or perhaps last weekend you took a walk in nature and, although for much of the time you were preoccupied with to-dos and work quandaries, there was also that blissful moment when you gazed out to take in the view and for just a few seconds became aware of a magnitude of quiet. Or perhaps you most recently found peace in that first mouthful of ice cream – not because it satisfied your taste buds but because, just for an instant, everything else stopped.

Can you recall a time, however recent or long ago, when you were hit by a sudden feeling of being both completely present and entirely connected to the people and experiences around you? If that's too strong, perhaps think back to a moment when you suddenly noticed a stillness — an OK-ness — without there being any particular reason why.

In all these examples, rest (stillness, silence. . . a harmonious no-thing) emerged only when everything else had faded away. That feeling of completeness – of everything being OK exactly as it is right now – was not brought into the experience but rather revealed itself only once everything else was gone. This quality of peace, it seems, is the only remaining constant when all other layers of our experience are removed. This is a wonderful thing to know. It is always present within us, even when we are experiencing great suffering. But it is also deeply frustrating, since we are unlikely to feel its presence if we are distracted by any other aspect of our experience.

Why we must stop trying to make ourselves restful

Rest enables us to connect more readily with the constant sense of OK-ness that is the backdrop of all experience, but we cannot enter rest with any conditions. As soon as we apply goals to rest, we turn it into a task, and it is no longer rest. For this reason, we must let go of any preconceived ideas we have about what rest is and what it should look like.

You have an opportunity here to surrender to the freedom that comes from not having to *know* how any of this works. You do not need to be an expert in meditation or an experienced yogi to 'do' anything we are sharing in this book – the point is: you need to do nothing.

And perhaps the greatest challenge of all will be to accept that this journey is not about helping yourself but about coming to the realisation that in spite of everything – all the suffering, all the stress, all the chaos, all the excitement, disappointments celebrations and grief – you exist from a place of constant, unshakable wholeness. There is part of you that doesn't need any help at all, ever.

> *— If you'd only stop looking, you'd see there is something fundamentally right with you.*

So, here we have yet another apparent contradiction: we want to emphasise that this is not a self-help book in its traditional form, yet we hope that this book will help you to see that part of you that needs no help. It is not a practical guide to positive thinking, a step-by-step route to achieving happiness, a collection of motivational mantras, a roadmap to realising your potential. But this is a self-help book in that it very much requires you to take on the idea that you are your best helper, and then see that it's not so much help that you need, but awareness, and then ultimately. . . that you *are* awareness.

But that's for you to find out, perhaps at the end of this journey.

The concept of helping yourself, or improving yourself, or bettering yourself (however you wish to label such a task) suggests you are somehow lacking. That you just need to do X, Y and Z, and bingo! New you. Whether that's a thinner, less anxious, better focused, more positive, less stress-heady version of yourself, most self-help books start with the assertion that you are not already OK. We, however, are suggesting that you are already OK, and that it might be that the very notion that you must *do* something to help you feel OK that is stopping you from feeling OK.

Again, we urge you to stop. Stop trying to help yourself. Or at the very least, take a rest from it.

ASK YOURSELF...

Do you 'do' anything in an attempt to feel more rested?
Can you see any contradiction in what you are doing? What leaves you feeling most rested?

Enquiry 2:
Why do you want to rest?

We so often fixate on what we want, and yet we so rarely ask ourselves why.

You might see how your answers are in conflict with the very nature of rest (and you might not).

Who's going to benefit from this rest? How? Does it matter if no one benefits? What is the point?

Is it OK to do something that is completely pointless?

Can anything be truly pointless?

There are endless paradoxes around the subject of rest. We can't do it, but we have to do it. We can't make ourselves do it, but it must be done. We cannot have the intention of it doing anything for us, but it will do everything for us. We cannot think our way into it, but by thinking about it when we are not doing it, we will become better at not-thinking our way into it.

But is this really that different from anything else? We learn to write not by reading but by writing; we learn to walk by walking, we learn to drive by driving, we learn to swim by swimming, we learn to love by loving. It is in the doing that we do, and the being that we are.

— Regardless of what you think you want, if you allow it, the rest will come, and the rest is easy.

- Prepare yourself for rest. You might want to sit, lie down, or you might want to stand and stare into space. Do whatever appeals. (You might also want to revisit Enquiry 1 on page 15)

- As you settle, you might notice your mind is racing. That's OK. Don't try to change anything. Stay with this for a few moments

- Now ask yourself what you hope to get out of all this – this resting, this stopping. What's driving you?

- Whatever your answer, now reflect on the possibility that restfulness is a quality within; not something to create but something to be recovered (or uncovered)

- What does this mean in terms of your motives for seeking out rest? Can you see any contradictions? It doesn't matter if you did (you cannot be 'wrong'). See if you can observe without criticism

- Continue to be still for a few moments, or minutes if time allows

- When you're ready to end the enquiry, have a stretch or take a deep breath

- As you consciously come out of rest, notice how you feel, and note any insights or important new understandings

- Take a moment to write down your reasons for rest. Reflect on them, read them back to yourself (put them on the fridge or on a sticky note)

- Remind yourself that whatever you thought, felt or experienced during this enquiry, was exactly as it should be

Learning to stop battling with yourself

Life can seem like a constant tug of war, with only ourselves on either side of the rope. The more we struggle, the more tension that builds, and, against our best efforts to sort ourselves out, we feel worse than before. We feel flawed, substandard, helpless, broken. We hope to introduce you to a new possibility and guide you just enough so that you might begin to see a truth that has been revelatory to many of us (a kind of 'quiet' movement if you will): that you cannot be broken. Fundamentally, deep down, you are already and always whole. Your deepest nature is wonderfully OK and absolutely doesn't need fixing. The deepest aspect of your self – this 'awareness' we've referred to – already knows this. In fact, to qualify that a little further, the deepest aspect of your self doesn't *know* anything; it is beyond knowledge, and it is beyond knowing – and that's the gift.

Concepts and theories aside, being told you are fundamentally OK when you feel anything but OK can feel like a slap in the face and far, far from the truth. Therefore, we'd like to ask that if you don't believe anything we have said so far, perhaps you could at least entertain it to be a possibility. For a short while, we ask you to just try on the idea that deep down you are fundamentally OK. Just *suppose* that in spite of it all, the very essence of your being wishes to change nothing about who you are or what you are going through right now. And then consider that your current beliefs about rest and how it should happen and how you should 'do' it might be exactly what is standing in the way of you connecting with this essence, and of you feeling rested.

If you can do this, then we can set about enabling you to experience it to be true. Our challenge as teachers is to convey something that allows the brain to ease off – to stop hunting for examples, facts and stats – and to step aside (do nothing!), so that that which lurks beneath can rise to the surface. We would be hypocrites if through this book we sought to instil a new set of beliefs in you, for it is beliefs that very often prevent us from seeing ourselves as fundamentally always OK.

Accepting that we rarely see ourselves clearly

We have two young children and therefore are often a little behind with the housework (this might be an understatement). There's a mirror on our landing that hangs high above our stairwell and in order to clean it we have to affix a feather duster to a broom handle and stand on tiptoe at the top of our ancient and precarious staircase. It's a monumental faff and one that sits fairly low on the priorities list, so as the months go by a very thin veil begins to cover the mirror that, even if we can't perceive it, means we can no longer see ourselves clearly. Now, if we left that dusting job for 40 years (entirely plausible) then we wouldn't be able to see ourselves clearly at all. Just a glimpse, an outline, a suggestion of who we are, with the gaps filled in by memories and ideas we already have about what we look like.

And that's how it is for most of us in terms of grasping our true identity. Our deeper nature is obscured by our other identities. Our stories of who we are on the surface, our thoughts, our feelings and bodily sensations all act like noise to cover up our deepest, unchanging nature. All of the things we believe we have to get done, everything we believe in and think we know to be true, and all our responses to the world with all its complexities – these are the things that lie in the way of something that underneath is always gleaming and clear, regardless.

We are not going to instruct you as to how best to dust your mirrors – that would go against the premise of this book, and as we have shared, we are not fans of dusting (or indeed any housework). Instead, we hope rather to lead you into an experience of seeing that you are the mirror, and feel the permanence of that fact regardless of how much dust you've gathered (or your penchant for cleaning).

We are a race of storytellers and belief-seekers, eager to find reasons and solutions at every turn, but this does not inhibit our ability to go beyond reason and take relief from the possibility that we don't have to have all the answers – or *any* answers, special techniques or particular insights to see our completeness. We don't, in fact, need anything.

Rest and thinking

Despite that thought seems to come as a constant stream of chat and insight, there are interludes between our thoughts. If we follow a train of thought to its conclusion, we will notice when a new one pops in, and sometimes we might notice a pause beforehand. Again, we might miss something here, believing that it is the conclusion of the thought that feels good (because we've worked something out), but really, the pleasure comes as much, if not more, from the fact that on concluding your thought, you are now not thinking at all. You're experiencing the ultimate holiday.

The challenge comes, then, that on realising this we can quickly jump onto the idea that if we could just stop thinking for five seconds, then we'd feel good. Once we begin to notice and enjoy these spontaneous moments of *not* thinking, we can't help but grasp for them. Our mind gets hold of the experience and wants more of it. It's like the mind knows that the spaces around thinking are really good but then thinks about them and spoils the whole show, like a child who's watching their favourite television programme but who gets so excited about it they can't stop talking all the way through.

We can't think ourselves into not thinking. At most, you might have 'held' your thoughts in the same way that you might hold your breath. There are activities that can 'control the mind' to a certain extent, such as concentration practices, but while it may be possible to create conditions for the mind to focus, such as reciting the same word over and over again (some people adopt a special word or mantra, but repeating 'fudge, fudge, fudge' might be as effective) or concentrating on a single point of focus (a candle is a popular one here, but a cupcake would do just as well – maybe a fudge one), we're still 'doing' something (not resting). We're still engaging in an activity. We may be experiencing a pause, but it's not a *natural* pause (we might even be supressing our mind, only to have it fight back harder later). There may be benefits to doing this, but it is not rest.

ASK YOURSELF

Is it possible to stop thinking? What happens when you try to stop your thoughts?

There are countless techniques designed to help you tame your mind, but it is not *necessary* to spend hours (or years) honing meditation techniques in order to experience a calm mind. It happens to all of us, often when we least expect it. In any case, the point is not to have a calm mind, but recognise the fact that we can and do have spontaneous moments when we are not thinking – when we are beyond thought.

A few seconds of not-thinking is all it takes for you to realise you are not your mind, and you can carry this realisation with you always. You might begin to sense that there is a great well of spacious, harmonious being already within you, whether it's through those first few moments when you wake up, a pause between thoughts, a middle-distance gaze or noticing how when you went to bed your natural sleep hormones pulled you gently from your thoughts and into a blissful state of being neither awake nor asleep.

As you gather more and more of these moments, you might begin to realise that there is something within you that is always calm, always as OK as you have ever felt. Crucially, this is not a feeling you have created, but rather you have *uncovered* it. It is never not there, even if it seems to 'disappear' behind the thoughts. Whether we are practised meditators who make a point of creating space for these pauses every day or a mere mortal who has never actively 'meditated', yet still has these pauses (because we all do all the time), the point to remember is that the relief comes not from the pause, but from what the pause reveals to us.

Rest is only truly restful if you recognise the significance of what lies behind the absence of everything.

(You might have to take a moment to think about that. . . but be sure to enjoy the pause at the end of the thought. . .)

Our expectations for rest might be in the way of us resting

For most of us, when we stop doing, we become more aware of our incessantly chattering mind. The more we notice this noise, the louder it becomes and the more stressed we might become about it not quieting down. . . and the further away we think we are from feeling calm. This is very often the experience of anyone trying meditation for the first time and why they might describe it as 'difficult'. But meditation is not something you make happen; it's what happens to you when everything else stops. For this reason, we are all natural meditators. It's not something we can be *bad at*.

Rest can only be found in letting things unfold exactly as they are, without expectations or conditions. If we expect rest to be a certain way, then we're looking for something. We're still *doing*.

For example, many of us turn to nature when we're feeling stressed out. A walk in the woods or a hike up the hill can offer a much-needed tonic to our ills, and they do very often leave us feeling the thing that we craved: a calmer, more at-ease mind. However, there will inevitably be times when we return from the great outdoors still grappling with a situation, or for whatever reason feeling tense, and we'll likely feel short-changed. 'It hasn't worked!' we bemoan, 'I don't feel any calmer!' But we're missing something here: when we take a walk or practise yoga or listen to our favourite soothing music, we may immediately be soothed and then be gratified by such an outcome, in the same way that we might watch a stand-up comedian to make ourselves laugh – we set a goal, took an action and experienced an outcome that pleased us. However, we are once again distracting ourselves and missing the main event. That is, we are not recognising the awareness that is witnessing everything unfold and has no investment in the outcome being one way or another.

An experience felt as a result of a deliberate action is only a sideshow. It is the rabbit coming out of the hat amidst a greater illusion. We are so fixated on the little magic trick, we may not notice that the stage on which it is being performed has vanished.

The statement that there is something directly in front of our nose, or to put it another way, that there's something hiding in plain sight, can be pointed to when we consider the phrase: *That which you are looking for, is that which you are looking from.*

Realising that what we are looking for is already here

There is no getting away from the fact that your attention loves 'stuff'. It loves objects that appear in its consciousness. This is one of the most confounding factors for anyone formally approaching meditation. They realise that their attention is constantly fixated on everything that passes by. From noticing sensations in their body, and then the images that might arise from them, or noticing the smell of dinner cooking and then the thought about what tomorrow might bring or the memory of what happened today at work. It goes on and on, and it seems never-ending.

Regardless of how much effort you put into calming your mind, your mind is never going to stop being your mind and doing what it wants to do: namely, controlling everything and working everything out. And even though your mind knows that its attempts to figure out how to make tomorrow's meeting go smoothly, for example, can only be a game (it knows it is impossible to foresee all factors involved in the situation at the time), it will continue to look for ways to control the situation and secure a pleasing outcome.

Your mind is just doing its job. It is the most loyal employee you're ever going to have, and rather than get frustrated with it for being so incredibly duty bound or chastising it for being in the way of you getting what you want (a moment's peace), you can take a step back and leave it to get on with things. When we do this, we allow for the possibility that while there is all this stuff going on 'in our heads', there is also something else that is not darting about, not planning, not worrying about anything and not even doing anything at all – it is just *allowing*. There is something beyond our thinking; something that is never distracted, and never bored. Something that has been here all your life.

It's here now, as you read these words. Aware, quiet, at peace, still and in need of absolutely nothing.

Therefore, if you find yourself declaring, 'I just can't switch off my mind,' (or, 'I had a stressful day off!') you might wish to remind yourself that this is an inconsequential observation and that you are by no means any further than anyone else from connecting with the quiet essence of awareness that lies beneath (and above and all around) all other aspects of your experience.

The trap might be in your trying to find it, but you never will, because your awareness isn't another object to find. It's not a thing, but that in which all things appear. It's not a place to get to or an experience to be created. Like trying to grab a handful of fine sand, the more you tighten your grip, the more it will slip from your fingers.

It cannot be found and it cannot be lost. It is always here.

> — *If rest is the ultimate act of doing nothing, then it has to involve doing nothing about the fact that your mind is not doing nothing.*

It's our hope that this is at once confounding and relaxing, and that as you read these words you feel relief from knowing that there's nothing you can do to get to this place of awareness – to that part of your experience that, regardless of what your mind and body are getting up to, is always OK. Your inner knowing, your deepest, wisest, most at-peace self is always there, and grappling over *how* you can find it (it's never lost) or complaining that you can't find it (it's always there) will only take you further away from realising that you are already it. You are always *being*.

However, we do appreciate that. . .

You can't pretend you don't want to feel rested and find peace

It is perhaps a cruel paradox that the more able you are to surrender to what is and give up the notion of having to do something to stop doing and start being, then the more likely you are to happen upon an experience of being. However, over time, your mind will get hold of this truth and bend it to its own agenda. The mind will start to say such things as, 'If I can give up my expectations then I'll get to this stillness and have an experience of peace and calm'. And just like that, you're back to watching the sideshow and not realising the main event is playing out right before your eyes.

We can't pretend our mind doesn't have this desire for results. There will always be part of you craving for direction and action to bring about a pleasing consequence. Thankfully, there are ways around this. For example, if your mind needs an aim to attach to the act of taking rest then it can be simply to find that which is already there, with no expectations for it looking one way or another.

If we can have a motive devoid of conditions and we free ourselves of the need for rest to look a particular way, we will find ourselves stepping back further into our unconditional self – our unbiased awareness. If we lay down for half an hour and get caught up in the noise of our mind then it doesn't matter, because we'll likely have also uncovered or remembered (albeit fleetingly) that part of our experience is doing very well (as always) without the need for a particular outcome – the part of us that is aware of all of this, but not *in* it.

The essence of our being doesn't require any conditions in order to *be*. If we can engage in the art of sitting quietly without trying to control the experience, or do anything, we'll have an even greater chance of glimpsing our essential self.

ASK YOURSELF

How often do you rest without having an expectation for how that period of rest will unfold and what the results of it might be?

Enquiry 3:
What happens if you turn your attention from thought to sensation?

Very rarely can we stop and immediately experience a quiet mind, but most of the time, as long as we remain still, our thoughts will settle and the noise diminish. However, there will be times when we enter thought loops that even after allowing them to whirl about just as they wish for some time, seem to gain momentum and grow even louder. Of course, you could just allow this to be the case, but you may alternatively like to try the following enquiry in which we explore the physical sensations in our body, as a kind of 'decoy mission'.

The enquiry involves performing a kind of 'attention scan' of our entire body. You might notice a tingling in the fingertips, an ache in the belly, a pain in the knee, lightness, heaviness, heat, cold or even that there is no particular sensation calling for attention. You might even become aware of a numbness. You can focus on a particular part of the body or, if you're feeling especially restless you can allow your attention to move. The key point with both is that you do not do anything with whatever you notice. You just watch.

By this process we switch our attention from thinking to sensations. If our thoughts were making us feel tense, we might now be experiencing that tension in the body instead. The 'issue' is now physical, not cerebral, and we're likely less concerned with wanting to work it out or come to a resolution. We're just observing it as physical sensation.

Something very interesting can happen at this point. When we allow ourselves to *feel* our tension (instead of thinking about it) and without intending to change it in anyway, that tension may begin to dissipate all of its own accord. There are, of course, lots of other possibilities. It might get more intense or shift and move around. What we are proposing is that you don't get too caught up in what's happening; that you instead, allow it to happen.

With this enquiry, you might experience your body's innate ability to bring itself back into balance (or 'harmony'), without 'you' having to do anything. That loop of worry, for example, has gone from the attention of your mind to a sensation in your body to being released, merely by you having allowed it to do so.

We can take this enquiry further by asking ourselves *where* is all this taking place? What is it that is holding all this experience? What is the backdrop to our thinking, our sensation and our allowing? Whether we're in a thought loop, scanning our body or glimpsing a stillness, how is the space in which this all unfolds affected? Does it ever change?

Typically, when we step back from any experience, we step into a spaciousness that knows no tension. We can remember that there's something right here (that's reading these words), that is aware of everything and has capacity for unconditional acceptance.

This enquiry can help us whenever we get caught up in refusing, resisting or running a commentary on our experience, so that we might glimpse at the space within which all our experience appears.

We might then find ourselves slipping effortlessly into that part of us that remains untouched and unbreakable.

- *Make yourself comfortable (sitting, lying; it doesn't matter)*

- *Notice your thoughts. Just watch. You might have a particularly busy mind, and that's actually beneficial to this enquiry. Allow it all to be just as it is for a few moments*

- *Now, turn your attention to sensation. Observe the overall feeling of your body. Perhaps you have an obvious niggle, or there's a familiar pain that presents itself to you. Perhaps you notice that you feel relaxed, or twitchy. However you are feeling, allow it to be*

- *If you're struggling to notice any sensation at all, see if you can draw your attention to how your body rests against the surface that's holding it*

- *Now, take your attention to your mouth. Notice the sensation of your tongue. Then the roof and sides of your mouth around it. Notice your jaw. Don't try to do anything about any tension or anything else you notice, just be with the sensation*

- *Now notice the sensation of your hands. Give up thinking about them; feel them. Notice the sensation of the palms. The feeling of air touching the skin. The feeling of the fingers and thumbs. Notice the right hand. Then the left hand. Then both hands at the same time*

- Feel your feet. Mentally scan every last element of your feet

- Once again, turn your attention to the parts of your body that are touching the surface that holds it

- Hang out here for as long as feels right – preferably minutes rather than moments

- Allow yourself to surface from this in a slow and leisurely way, noticing how you feel in body and mind

Why Are We Restless?

Everywhere we look, we're faced with messages of self-improvement, self-mastery, self-betterment and acquisition. Wherever you are in life, whether you've just landed your first job or are a multi-millionaire, you'll always want more. Whereas on the one hand we are urging you to see that at your core, you need for nothing, there is also a dance to be done as a human, that involves experiment, creation, exploration and, certainly, acquisition. Let's call this the desire to *become*. There's nothing wrong with it, and indeed, you'll spend most of your life 'becoming': growing older, wiser, learning from mistakes, becoming more accomplished at being a parent or a leader or a gardener or cook, or whatever specialism appeals to you or whatever role you find yourself in whether you planned it or not. Nobody spends their entire life 'being'. When we contemplate that we can both 'be' and 'become', there is less of a tension between the pull of desires and the relief from recognising that you do not need your desires to be fulfilled (beyond basic requirements for human survival, of course). You do not have to choose one over the other.

What we're proposing when we talk about 'being' is to take time in your life and even more importantly, adopt an attitude or mental position, in which you can let go of desires and the desire to control any aspect of your experience. The more frequently you do this not-doing, the more likely you are to glimpse the contented wholeness of your deepest being, and the more that aspect of your being will permeate through all other aspects of your experience.

What's interesting, is that once you've gained access to this restful being within you, there's less of a need to carve out times of 'actively not doing'. This *being* accompanies you in to the rest of your life, and you will likely feel overwhelmed, tired and cut off from yourself less and less. The need to escape to an island of rest is not an uncommon image many people discuss. While that island might be necessary to begin with, ultimately this restful place is found and stabilised within you, and informs the rest of your life.

Rest takes us to arguably the richest and most insightful place we can come to in our lives, it's just that the act that leads us to this insight looks and feels like a dead end. This is a good thing to remember next time you feel like you are staring down a dead end.

Why do we forget that rest is elusive?

When you take a deeper look at the moments when you arrive at a rested experience, they are with surprising regularity magical. Often, it is our happiest moments and our most endearing memories that equate to rest. That unexpected breath-taking sunset we were able to share with our beloved. That moment we lay down in the dew-ridden grass, looked up at the stars and realised we could only ever know one thing: that life is mysterious (and yet we still asked, *what's it all about?*). The time we took a train journey and fell inexplicably into a deep sense of ease and relaxation, even though our life was busy and tiring. Those times when we fall into hysterical laughter with friends and behind the giggles we also feel an indescribable sense of belonging, not only to those friends but also to our entire lives. These peak experiences are born out of no-thing – we didn't think them into happening, they weren't an event we were able to orchestrate, and often the fact that we don't foresee these experiences is what makes them all the more joyful. And yet, we continue to live our lives chasing these moments, trying to work them out and trying to recreate them, forgetting that they happened to us in the moment we *stopped trying to do anything*.

So, why do we forget? Why is it so hard to trust that we do not need to do anything to experience these moments of what some people describe as 'bliss'?

One challenge that we all face is how our mind takes hold of these experiences. As you may have noticed, you very rarely have a single line of thought about anything. For example, if you're planning something for the future there might be part of you that feels fear, while another part has a sense of excitement, and there will also be an aspect of you that would rather sort out the kitchen cupboard than go over everything again, and so on. With blissful moments, while there will be part of us that recalls them as free and full and happy memories, our 'thinking' brain – that part of us that likes to plan, orchestrate successes and avoid failure – will grasp the experience and try to work it out ('*it happened because of this*', '*it means that*', etc.).

> — *The restful experience itself goes against the very nature of the story-telling mind.*

When we rest, our thoughts tend to quieten down, or we might loosen our identity with them as we fall into a more daydream-like quality of being. And it is this looseness that feels like a threat to that part of us that likes to know what's going on, that likes to get places and is often (if not always) looking out for the next thing. The prospect of stopping and doing nothing, of resting, can set off alarm bells in our head. This is why, although it sounds ridiculous, doing nothing can seem very hard – there is an aspect of our self that is incredibly resistant to it. When we set about resting, we often start to feel far more rest*less* than before we set about resting. Typically, we give up resting because we deem it to be 'not working' – we chastise our active minds for having taken us away from the possibility of resting.

So, what must we do about this?

The answer is, as you might have guessed, nothing. You rest by doing nothing, and this means doing nothing about the fact that you don't seem to be resting.

There is nothing 'wrong' with any of your resistance to rest and, interestingly, it doesn't stop you from resting, as long as you don't try to do anything about the resistance. You do not have to resist the resistance. As you embark on a moment of rest (a conscious 'stopping'), you may well become frustrated, annoyed and confused, and you may feel more restless than when you were actively 'doing' something. But this is OK because just as black needs white and hot needs cold and up needs down, rest needs restlessness. It's all part of the journey. . .

Restlessness is not stopping you from resting

When we declare ourselves in need of rest, what we are essentially saying is that we need to stop. We recognise a need to remove distraction and activity from our experience so that we may find some kind of quiet. However, we often find distraction and frustration along the way, and indeed, we very often fail to feel rested regardless of our trying to create the conditions in which we believe rest will come. We make an effort to schedule-in activities that we believe are restful, rather than face the fact that what we really need to do is nothing.

The tricky thing about rest is that regardless of how much we need it, we cannot *make* it come. We cannot force ourselves to rest and trying to rest will rarely land us in a place anywhere near rest-town (trying implies effort, whereas rest is an anti-effort kind of a gig). What's more, we expect the journey to rest-town to be a peaceful one, but it isn't always. To enter a state of true rest – to find that place of absolute quiet – we must be prepared to venture through unsettled waters and come face-to-face with our chattering mind. It's all-too-easy to assume that a noisy mind is a symptom of somehow 'failing' to rest, when it's very often a sign that you are well on your way to resting.

ASK YOURSELF

Spend a few moments observing the chatter of your thoughts. How did it make you feel? Did anything change in the way you perceive your thoughts?

We have all this to face on top of the fact that we live in an action-obsessed society, where effort and perseverance are considered not only vital (to success, happiness and health) but also, somehow, inherently virtuous.

Rest, in its truest sense of doing absolutely nothing – and definitely not doing any rest-based activities (what?) and definitely not photographing any of it and sharing it on social media – has completely gone out of fashion, and so in this way, what we are proposing via this book is something very anti-culture, and therefore, we like to think, deliciously rebellious.

Do you think it's OK to do nothing?

Many of us live with the belief that in order to be rewarded with something good we must first endure something difficult. We must work hard to get the things we want. We feel a sense of achievement if we put ourselves through a punishing workout, slog away at a work project, or even endure pain. We see difficulty as a precursor to the reward. When something good appears to land in our laps we feel suspicious, and sometimes even ashamed. We might also begrudge those to whom this happens.

We are encouraged to have goals, to reach for the stars, to strive, push and plough on, even when we're desperate for relief. If we're not working hard at something, we're not playing the game and we're letting the team down. We even ask, 'Keeping busy?' as a means to enquire after someone's wellbeing.

ASK YOURSELF

Do you ever feel guilty for taking time out? If so, where does that feeling come from – pressure on yourself, others, society?

We are taught from a young age that hard work reaps reward and that graft and application are precursors to success and happiness (precarious words in themselves). Many schools in the UK and US now make a point of praising students for their effort and resilience as much, if not more, than the outcome of their work. The idea is to take the focus off inherent ability and encourage children to see they are limited only by their *attitude* to work – that talent is not the key to success, but rather effort and focus are. It's an approach that forgets that it is impossible to quantify effort. If you're working hard at something because you are enjoying it, is that effort? Will you be praised? If you're working hard at something you don't enjoy, should you be praised more? If a child finds something easy and fun at school that most other children find difficult and boring, should that child do more or less of that thing?

You've probably heard the saying, 'Choose a job you love, and you will never have to work a day in your life'. It encapsulates the point that when pleasure and effort are combined, then the feeling of anything having been hard work is diminished. So why are we so intent on focusing on the 'hard work' aspect of life, than the pleasure?

It's impossible to have a clear answer to that question. To put effort at the centre of an education model is perhaps a decent way to ensure all children are treated equally and see themselves as such, but perhaps it also teaches them to undervalue – or worse, be apprehensive about – play, experiment, daydreaming, messing around, lolling about: times when we discover our pleasures, passions and our peace. And vitally, it is during these effortless downtimes that we are most likely to have remarkable insight and clarity.

— *Sometimes doing nothing is the most productive thing we can do.*

We've all experienced those *aha*! moments, when solutions jump out of nowhere when we weren't even thinking about the problem. You'd set your mind to the task and kept going around in circles and then only as you had given up on the problem and given yourself a rest from the issue, perhaps turning your attention to something less 'heady' (the washing up, brushing your teeth) did the insight appear.

Apparently, when Einstein found himself feeling dozy, he would sit in a comfortable chair with a pen between his hands, knowing that he would drop it at just the point before nodding off and catch himself in that magic pre-sleep state where he might have the chance to capture insights or solutions that his awake-brain was not able to figure out. Similarly, Edgar Allan Poe talked of the 'fancies' that would come upon him, 'only when I am on the brink of sleep, with the consciousness that I am so'. The German chemist Kekulé reported discovering or 'seeing' the ring-like structure of benzene amidst a daydream, only to later formulate his discovery. Lewis Carol's *Alice in Wonderland* is rumoured to be an attempt to capture one such waking dream.

Can you recall a time when you had a flash of insight 'out of nowhere'? How did it come about? What did it feel like?

Evidently, these moments when our brains are quiet and we've ceased trying to figure anything out are vital to our ability to find answers and be creative. However, this is a very difficult concept to convey because setting about a moment of rest with the intention of getting anything out of it may well hinder your ability to rest, and yet if you manage to take a moment of proper rest, you will probably get an enormous amount out of it. The key is to separate intention from influence: you can approach rest with the intention of gaining insight, though you must relinquish any desire to control what that insight might be or how it will come. As soon as we try to have influence on our experience of rest, we are adding to our experience, not taking away, and it is the taking away that allows insight to appear. When Einstein sat in his chair, he may have had something of a shopping list of requirements, but crucially he knew he couldn't take this into the rest-state with him. He knew that a raw openness to whatever may come – an approach of allowing over controlling – was the only way to be.

This complete surrendering is a difficult pill to swallow, and it is a contradictory pill because of course – *of course* – you want there to be an outcome to your rest. You want to feel rested, clearer, brighter, and maybe even gain some insight, and you itch to find a way to guarantee such an outcome. It seems as though effort, planning and measurable output are the more reliable means to achievement and so we opt to invest in these over rest. We believe that effort and focus will be rewarded because the alternative seems preposterous – that good fortune will land in our laps if we only relaxed, took time to be, and allowed output (ideas, inventions, opportunities) to present themselves to us.

The notion that you'll never be the best you can be unless you work hard to be better than you are right now is a shocking insult to the amazing, creative, unique being you already are, a being whose objective in life might not be to 'win' at everything, but to be engaged and delighted by, and kind to, the world around them, with all its gifts, surprises and mind-blowing mysteries. This does not mean you have the wrong mindset, or are lazy, but maybe just a little less preoccupied with that which you do not have right now. We are distracted by the 'must dos' when so many of the must-dos are conceptual.

That said, the washing up does actually have to be done, the bins do have to go out, the laundry pile won't sort itself out, and we all need to earn a living somehow – and of course we must recognise that there is a difference between inaction as a result of despondency and inaction through honouring the importance and possibilities of rest.

We are not advocating a giving up of all doings. More, we are urging you to see the value of doing nothing alongside all your doing, and see how it will perhaps make all the doing all the more ease-filled. And then, who knows, with a new-found ease, creative insight, a delightful lightness to your work, you might achieve something utterly amazing. . . or you might not. And that's OK too.

Lifestyle versus real-style

If we are so unlikely to glimpse our innate 'OK-ness' by effort, if we don't have to try to be aware, because we always are aware, then why do we put so much effort into creating a lifestyle that we believe represents balance, wellbeing and self-care?

We are bombarded with information and images regarding how to lead a balanced and healthy lifestyle, and it all looks very complicated (though, admittedly, rather pretty). To be healthy and well has become 'aspirational' – a buzzword used to describe goods and lifestyles that are out of reach, either because they are too expensive or require an inordinate amount of commitment and effort. Many brands, including people who consider themselves brands, aspire to be aspirational; it is seen as a positive thing. However, it's an approach that relies on convincing audiences that a healthy, balanced lifestyle is available only to those willing to put enough effort in to achieving it. It enables a few at the top to preach down to the masses. It sets most of us up as losers but dangles just enough of a carrot to keep us fantasising about a future in which we might be a better version of the person we are now, with the fit body, a rainbow nutrient diet, glowing skin, luxury fitness clothes and the right kind of 'fierce' attitude to cling on to it all.

(It is ironic how many aspirational brands on social media present themselves as advocates of the 'I am enough,' concept – the yogini with her leg stretched at angles at which Mother Nature would flinch, telling you that you are perfect just as you are. . . but perhaps not as perfect as she is.)

You might find relief in the possibility that doing nothing is as, if not more, likely to make you feel good about yourself as doing something. Though equally, perhaps it's an unsettling concept: it removes the fantasy future and puts everything within your reach. If we are already OK, then what are we to do about all these feelings of lack and inadequacy? Are they not going to get better? To go away?

If we can entertain the idea that feeling whole, balanced and complete is not a matter of attainment or achievement, but a matter of allowing ourselves to be with who we are when all these things are stripped away, we can see ourselves more clearly. We might be kinder to ourselves, we might discover aspects of ourselves that surprise us. We might become more playful in our choices. We might make choices most in-line with our inherent preferences, or simply to experiment without agenda or pressure, with gentleness and intrigue. We're not trying to 'get anywhere' but because we are alive and engaged with the world we are still travelling through life. We are still changing, learning and growing, but we are also honouring the completeness of who we already are.

ASK YOURSELF

*Is there anything you are doing in your life right now
that you believe will 'make you a better person'?
What do you hope to change about yourself?*

In order to feel better about who you are and what you are doing right now you need nothing.

There's no food you can eat, exercise routine you can perform, outfit to wear, toxic friends to unfriend, work to quit, that will leave you feeling as good about yourself as if you took some time out each day to sit and be (or stand and be – however you are inclined to stop) and be reminded of that which lies behind all your experience: stillness, awareness and absolute acceptance of who you are right now.

The 'rest' trap we have today is that there are countless activities that might appear to be rest inducing, but rarely involve rest in its purest form. They have just enough of a 'relax' element to make us feel as though we are resting, but they have enough purpose to reassure us we are not wasting our precious free time. They leave us with something to talk about – something to photograph, share or even boast about. But they are all ways to add to our experience rather than take away.

Whoever you are and however you live, your ability to rest is the same as anyone else. Rest needs nothing; it is not a lifestyle choice.

Rest, when it's happening (although it is the happening of nothing) is totally unproductive, and this can be a terrifying prospect for many of us. How often have you woken up at the weekend with no plans and on the one hand felt relieved by the prospect but on the other a little edgy? How many times have you gone on holiday with absolutely nothing on your itinerary? How many times have you thought about trying out meditation or even just taking a nap but have chosen instead to do something that will bring about immediate results? The prospect of doing nothing comes with all sorts of guilt and fear, even when we feel our being crying out for absolute stillness. We still resist for fear something will slip, that our future will be negatively impacted by our decision to stop or our fantasy future will be delayed by our inaction.

ASK YOURSELF

When you imagine yourself doing absolutely nothing, how do you feel? What do you think might be the 'cost'?

For some of us, the only time we don't feel guilty for not doing anything is when we are ill. Suddenly, we have a reason to completely down tools. On these days, we are allowed to not 'seize the day' and instead recuperate (so that we can get back to being busy again. . .).

In many ways, we are deeply afraid of simplicity and ease, even though for many of us, our fantasy future features both these things in abundance.

Enquiry 4:
What can be missing from no-thing?

If you want to feel rested, then it's hard not to start thinking about what you need to change in your life to allow that to happen. You might determine that rest will only come if certain conditions are met, and so you might start rejecting anything that doesn't fit the picture of rest you had imagined and you go looking for conditions that do. 'If I could just get some proper quiet then I'd be able to really settle in to this rest thing they keep talking about,' or, 'If I could be completely and perfectly comfortable, then I could relax. . .'

What we'd like you to enquire about here is the possibility that the thing you are looking for is already within you, and it's something that is beyond peace, that's already relaxed, that is already *whole*. You don't need to learn how to focus your mind or use a fancy meditation stool or create a blissfully quiet environment to discover it. What we are pointing to is beyond all of those pre-conditions. It is beyond *any* condition.

Whether you have experienced this as true or not, it can be an interesting experiment to just try this attitude on. Your mind will forever wish to reject the notion that everything is OK, just as it is – it will not accept that you are already perfect. It cannot, because its job is to find ways to make things better and safer and bigger, etc. The only part of you that *can* take this stance of perfection is the part of you that knows it to be true – that quiet, essential 'you' that is simply watching all of this carrying on.

Adopting the possibility that you need nothing to rest helps us call out all of the ways in which we might feel we are creating less than perfect circumstances for resting ('I can't switch my mind off!') or that life is in the way of those perfect circumstances ('The fridge won't stop buzzing!'). If we can see how these might be distractions, and we become aware of them as such, we might then notice that they appear within our own quiet, watchful sentience. We can notice that everything we are thinking and feeling about rest, and the conditions in which we think it might need to come, is all happening within the deeper experience of our rested self.

- *Apply everything you've learnt, through trial and error, about rest so far. Do whatever works for you to get still and comfy*

- *Remind yourself that during this enquiry you will notice 'imperfections' in your experience of rest and that, as much as you are able to, you are to surrender to them. This is an invitation to give up the need for perfect circumstances*

- *Settle yourself, perhaps observe your breath for a few moments, notice the sensations in your body. Just watch and be with everything just as you are and just as everything around you happens to be*

- *Spend a few minutes just 'being' in this way*

- *Now, we invite you to look out for a perfection that already exists: when you become preoccupied or feel something to be 'imperfect' during this period of rest, are you also then able to* notice a contrasting quality? What is there behind the distraction?

- Keep falling into that space behind the distractions and sensing into a quality that might always be still, whole, complete, perfect and not bothered about anything. This is not something you have to find; it's already here. It's watching you reading these words

- See if you can continue to fall back in to it, effortlessly

- Rest in this 'completeness' – this 'perfection' – for as long as you like. Indulge yourself

- When you're ready, bring your focus back to your body and to your breath

- Now consciously let go of everything you experienced during the enquiry – as we go about our daily lives, we may not feel this sense of 'perfection' and 'wholeness', and that's OK

- But we might find we put less pressure on ourselves to be perfect

Is life complicated, or do we complicate life?

With very few exceptions we approach most aspects of our lives, including rest, as a task to be taken on, figured out, improved and refined. We're constantly drawing up to-do lists (if not literally then metaphorically), setting goals and nagging and berating ourselves over every detail of our existence and then asking *why* about everything. *Why* can't I hold down a relationship? *Why* am I so shy? *Why* do I hate every job I take on? *Why* do I get so frustrated with my children? And then we try to figure out how to make it all better: '*How* can I be a better partner?', '*How* can I be more confident?', *How* can I be more patient with my children?' '*How* can I find a career I love?'.

We're becoming as exhausted by our inner dialogues as we are by the practical comings and goings of our external lives. All the while, we believe that this is how it's supposed to be: things are supposed to be hard, that we must be putting effort into improving ourselves and understanding ourselves and getting to the bottom of everything we are because as we are right now, we are not doing enough. We are not enough.

— Peace, ease and simplicity will come, when we get it done.

— But, we never get it done.

— Nobody ever gets it done.

Diet is a particularly obvious example of how we constantly try and fail to engage in a programme of 'self-care' and become exhausted by our own self failings and then try even harder to fix our failings, and so continues the loop of trying and failing and believing that the resolution will come tomorrow, once we've realigned our efforts and armed ourselves with the right kind of knowledge and *tried harder*. How many times in your life have you embarked on a healthy eating regimen, cleared out the cupboards of anything 'naughty' only to, over a few weeks, find yourself somehow exactly back where you started, munching on double-chocolate cookies and feeling confused and depressed by your inability to look after yourself? Even though you enjoyed the healthy eating phase, for one reason or another it didn't stick. Life happened. You, without even realising, made a series of choices that took you right back to where you were before. And so, you plot yet another way to 'sort yourself out'.

De-cluttering is another example. We very often go through our wardrobes and cupboards, creating huge bag-loads of clothes, books and other paraphernalia that we gleefully whisk off to the charity shop feeling both good about the deed and refreshed about our now full-only-of-stuff-that-brings-us-joy home, but a few months later the cupboards are overflowing with junk once more and we're sitting at our desk wearing a grubby old sweatshirt that may bring us warmth but certainly not joy. At no point did we say to ourselves, 'I miss being surrounded by stuff. I'm going maximalist!' Instead, it's more likely we just got distracted, slipped into old habits, turned our attention to other things, or, even for only a moment, just stopped caring so much.

We see various aspects of who we are and what we do to be in need of an overhaul, and then typically we take on someone else's ideas of the best way to live, and then struggle — because they inevitably will not be in synch with our natural inclinations. We very rarely approach those things we wish to change about ourselves with any kindness, patience or even just openness. We're more likely to 'tackle', 'control', 'deny', 'fix' a 'problem' than just *be* with it.

There are countless solutions to a whole host of 'problems' out there, but they are only ever a mixture of someone else's definition of what the problem is and therefore what might be the way around it. There is no prescription to remedy your own behaviour because all your behaviours have meaning of relevance only to you, and none of them are in themselves 'bad' or indeed 'failures'. You might see what this behaviour is really all about by stopping and observing it without any 'shoulds,' 'coulds' or 'what-ifs.'

> — *The task is not to search for answers, but to allow for awareness.*

It's a simple proposition that demands you give up trying to 'do' anything before first simply *being* with your situation — without having to 'figure' it out or analyse anything in any way. And it's a very positive proposition because it places all the power within you. Crucially, it involves, in the first instance, *doing nothing*.

Which is so far from what we are led to believe is the best way to 'be a better version of ourselves'.

We're encouraged to think that feeling better about ourselves is an enormous undertaking typically involving complicated methods or transformation. Whether it's by marketing and advertising, media and pop culture, or even our parents or teachers, we have become convinced that life is riddled with obstacles that require hard work or precise techniques to be overcome. We learn to believe that life inevitably involves a war on those aspects of ourselves that we believe are failing us. We must fight to win. We must *make* ourselves to change.

It's an aggressive mindset, and it's exhausting.

There are many forces at work here, but an obvious one is the objective to profiteer from our feelings of failure and lack: for example, the more a company can convince you that you have a problem (a cold, weight gain, sleep issues), and the more serious they can make out the problem to be, the more complicated they can make their solution appear (the product) and the more likely you are to believe in its efficacy to eliminate the problem, the more willing you are to pay a great deal for it.

A lot of power in the world is gained by convincing people that they need a lot of help. That they need to force themselves to change. That they should *keep going* until they've changed. What we're proposing is that you should stop everything (and rest) first, and then see what changes.

We don't want to get all conspiracy theory on you here, because there are some aspects of our experience as humans that really are complicated and really do require skills outside of our own capability to help bring us back to good health – or back to balance – not feeling overwhelmed by anything. We hope common sense makes it clear what these particular challenges are: a plaster for a cut, a vaccine for a specific illness, a cookie for a sudden urge to munch on something sweet and crumbly. However, it is for those more nebulous areas of difficulty that we are very often encouraged to believe the solution is to invest in something unusual or complicated or time-consuming and expert.

And, we're not saying that there aren't methods, resources and individuals out there that offer wonderful remedies and insight. There are. We are, right now, suggesting that stopping, doing nothing, might, without effort, bring about the very shift you were frantically searching for.

When we are feeling stressed, for example, we might be tempted to seek out a remedy for our 'condition,' and we will soon find countless solutions to choose from, from the mundane to the ridiculous. Just as is the case with effort, it's hard to measure stress (one person's 'stress' might be another's 'mild frustration'), and it's hard to measure how much a particular remedy has made a difference, but fundamentally the solutions we are presented with all-too-often involve adding something *into* our experience rather than taking something away to leave us with space (even if that 'addition' is taking on the task of decluttering or detoxing).

The possibility that what we need most when we are feeling overwhelmed is nothing is something that is overlooked as we invest more of our precious time in shopping around for solutions. Furthermore, although we recognise that we must perhaps 'do' less, we often deem this to be out of the realms of possibility. The simple truth is that we might just feel a little less stressed if we took a few moments (right now!) and did nothing, allowing the brain and body to rebalance themselves (which they are very able to do). This simple act, that takes barely any time from your day, is something so many of us resist in the belief that its simplicity is an indication of its ineffectiveness.

The belief that we require something complicated and difficult to find rest is very often the one thing in the way of us simply, and even sometimes easily, resting.

Enquiry 5:
How are you breathing?

How you breathe affects how you feel, and how you feel affects your breath. The simple act of observing your breath can change both how you feel and how you breathe. This is a superpower we all have.

The human nervous system has two essential systems, one of stimulus and one of rest and relaxation. Both are autonomous, meaning they don't require control. They are influenced by how much stimulus we take in and how much rest we engage in. It's an important and fascinating consideration, especially if we look at the levels of rest versus stimulus we currently have in our society today.

The *rest* part of our nervous system (called the parasympathetic nervous system) is largely responsible for healing, health, digestion and releasing tension. We activate this part of our nervous system by taking rest and, to some degree, when we breathe out.

When we breathe in, generally speaking, we receive a stimulatory tone, and when we breathe out, our nervous system is calmed. We've heard of plenty of people who have greatly improved their health from learning to either breathe in more if they needed energising, or breathe out more if they needed relaxation. However, very rarely are people taught how best to breathe for them, and practising breathing in a group might mean you take on a process that is totally ill-fitting for you. If you're already experiencing a lot of tension and stress, you don't want to do a lot of intense breathing in. . . you might blow up (metaphorically, of course).

So, we can't prescribe a breathing practice for you, but we can work with observing what already happens in your body.

When there's a balance between stimulus and relaxation, your body moves towards optimal regulation. The thing to remember is that when your body rests, *it looks after itself*. You do not need to do anything (apart from nothing).

If you took half an hour to simply stop and do nothing (see Enquiry 1 on page 15), you will likely notice that by the end, your out-breath will have become noticeably longer. Without you having done anything, your body has set about the task of restoring itself. This has not happened by effort, or indeed by magic, but it is your body's natural balancing act. (If your out breath didn't lengthen during Enquiry 1 then you might like to experiment with *Enquiry 3: What happens if you turn your attention from thought to sensation?* on page 46).

Either formally or informally, you will at some point in your life have turned your attention to your breath. This might have been as complicated as performing some kind of convoluted sequence of breathing, counting, holding your breath and using a visualisation, or as simple as taking a deep breath before asking someone out on a date. In this enquiry, we're simply going to watch our breath, albeit through a kind of mental magnifying glass:

– *Set yourself up for a few moments of doing nothing. You can sit or lie down, just make yourself comfortable and remove as many distractions as possible*

- Begin by simply observing how you are breathing right now. It might take you a little while to do this without interfering with the breath. Very often, once we watch our breath, we start to alter it even when we think we are not. Just sit (or lie) and be with your breath for a few moments

- Now, notice the out-breath, and then the in-breath. How does one feel in relationship to the other? Take your time. It will likely take a few minutes for you to notice anything in particular

- Keep going, keep resting, keep breathing (very important that you keep breathing. . .)

- Stay present with your breath for a few minutes. Just watching and allowing

- Keep going. If you have the urge to stop, see if you can keep going just a little longer (gently, no punishing here, please)

- When you feel it is time to resurface, pay final close attention to the relationship between your in-breath and out-breath. Has anything changed?

- If nothing changed, then nothing changed. You still got to take rest!

- Gently move your body and allow your attention to wander away from the breath (if it wants to. . .)

Rest forces you to be with yourself

Resting requires no skill and no knowledge. Anyone can rest. However, it does require us to surrender any desire to distract ourselves from ourselves.

Typically, stopping means we must face the clamour of our minds or be hit by a feeling we hadn't paid any attention to for some time. Proclaiming yourself incapable of switching off might be an excuse to avoid facing your inner dialogue (and everything else 'in there'), as much as an excuse for the fact that you do not have any trust in, or do not wish to see, what lies behind the noise – that essence of you that is left when everything else is gone. While part of you might know that you are just as capable as anyone else of switching off, you might also be too afraid to do it, don't fully see the value in doing it, or don't want to do it in case the 'you' that you do see when you switch off has no value to you (or scares you).

We've had all these feelings about rest, too. We've had that fear of being 'alone with our thoughts' – forgetting, as always, that between the thoughts, and behind the thoughts, is our unwavering home ground of simply *being*.

— *When we rest, we cannot hide from ourselves, and only when we see ourselves can we make friends with ourselves.*

You could take this in a very literal sense. If you are prepared to take on some of the ideas and practices that are to come in this book, you'll begin to fall in love with yourself (or to be more accurate, to see that you have always been in love with yourself and everything that ever was and is around you). You'll see that when you're constantly running on empty, frazzled and always looking for the next buzz, you're in many ways also running away from being with yourself. You're distracting yourself from yourself. You might think you're avoiding boredom or investing in a future that has everything just as you want it to be, but you are also avoiding being with yourself as you are right now. You are not giving yourself the time of day in the belief that you have better, more important things to do (such as fixing yourself).

If this has a ring of truth for you, perhaps you might want to ask how others might feel if you treated them the way you treat yourself. . .

Do you have time to be with yourself?

All the little decisions we make throughout the day about what to do next and what has to be done and what we think we want to do usually lead us to at no point taking the decision to rest. Day after day can go by in this way, and sometimes even years go by without us taking a deliberated moment to stop and be.

However, after reading this book, we hope you don't feel that you must somehow create a programme of rest. If you start making rest a 'do' on your to-do list then you are, albeit unintentionally, actively seeking to add more into your experience. Rest requires you follow no schedule, recite no mantras, aim for no goals, stick to no agenda.

> — *With rest, you are off the hook. Always.*

We've shown you that whether you knew it or not, you catch glimpses of your deepest, always-at-rest self throughout the day, every day: those moments when you first wake up, the pause between thoughts, those middle-distance gazes that feel inexplicably restorative, to name a few of the unnameable. But are these 'mini-awakenings,' enough?

Is there somehow a way to do more of nothing?

Do you need more or less to see, and remember, that at your core, you are whole – you are at peace?

How do you get more of less without doing more of less?

It's quite a conundrum.

Each day does present more opportunities than we realise to catch a glimpse of this consciousness – this restful awareness – and the likelihood is that from having simply considered this possibility, you will notice these moments more, and remember them. It goes without saying that this is not something you can force, but simply be open to. Once we start to see that being has as much value as doing, we might find ourselves less resistant to situations in which we might do nothing.

We know that the times when you need rest the most are those that allow for it the least. Often when we have 'too much' to do, we prioritise the doing stuff over the being stuff, because we simply don't have time to stop.

Very often the first thing we remove from our schedules when we are feeling time pressure are those things that leave us feeling spacious and nourished – cooking wholesome meals, taking long walks, relaxing with friends. We deem looking after ourselves in this way as a luxury we can no longer afford.

Unconscious neglect

Perhaps in such times we must ask ourselves what life has come to if we are actively choosing to *not* look after ourselves.

Of course, that's the problem – we do so without realising. We very rarely 'actively' choose to not look after ourselves. We generally neglect ourselves by accident and slowly over time. When work pressure takes over, for example, we don't consciously think, 'I will now eat pies and give up Pilates so that I can focus on my career', although that might be what actually happens. Similarly, if we have been through a particularly bad relationship breakup, it's not that we actively choose to overlook our physical health but more that we are so distracted by our grief that it doesn't feature strongly enough on our radar.

The problem with being human is that we are very easily distracted and then also firmly hardwired into certain behaviours in ways we can't even begin to see. We spend a great deal of our lives trying to coach ourselves into giving up old habits and creating new ones, and then failing at both and berating ourselves, and so we go on. We are in a constant state of struggle and become increasingly befuddled by our own behaviour. We ask ourselves why we are doing things we don't want to do. Is it that we actually want to do them? How can there be part of us that wants to do one thing but does the exact opposite? How can we have the intention but the opposite action? How can we *forget* to do the things we want to do for ourselves? Who's in control here?

We are in an unending cycle of distraction and frustration that is perhaps becoming worse. Smartphones are a key player in this cycle today; whether we're using them to chat, shop, research or take pictures, we've become unable to put them down for any significant length of time – even when we *want* to put them down, we often can't. At first it seems more relaxing to scroll through our phones than to witness what happens in our heads when we stop.

If you imagine your mind is a kitten (so cute!) we've got to a point where we are dangling wool in front of it for hours on end, without giving the poor little thing any opportunity to go lie in the sun. That kitten has become overly tired and frantic.

It's not just the amount of time we're using our phones, but that we choose to pick them up when we otherwise would have had a moment to do nothing – those few moments when you're in a café with a good friend/necessary enemy, and they pop to the bathroom, or those minutes when your toddler's fallen asleep in the car and you want them to have just a little bit longer. With no one to talk to and nothing much to be doing, our minds can throw up some bonkers stuff. This can be disconcerting, and so rather than face the chatter, we hop online and have a sniff about for something interesting and inevitably fall down various rabbit holes as the next virtual thing promises to be more interesting than the last, and before you know it, you've read the entire internet and, amazingly, feel emptier than before.

Although on one level we know that having a new message on our preferred social media platform is unlikely to be of serious conse-quence, the fact that the 'new message' icon is red makes it very hard for us to ignore the pull to read it immediately. The colour red draws our attention and operates as a mark of urgency and importance and the orchestrators behind those platforms employ such tactics to manipulate our behaviour and pull us into engage-ment. We feel we must see how many new 'likes' we have, how many 'shares', how many comments, etc. It temporarily feels life affirming, when in most instances the content is trivial and often irrelevant to our actual 'real life'. Social media offers a good example of how easily we can be side-tracked from the reality and value of our own experience of life. A few minutes online can leave us feeling drained and confused about who we are.

What we're doing in these precious could-be-quiet moments when we pick up our phones is denying our minds the opportunity to release some noise, and blocking any chance of us experiencing the benefits of the aftermath: peace, flashes of unexpected insight, silence.

Just like our kitten, the human being's nervous system needs both rest and engagement. Taking in a constant stream of 'more' can be overwhelming, yet, paradoxically, when our minds are that full, the last thing we want to do is stop.

We can't tell you *how* to stop or present a list of should and shouldn'ts when it comes to how you use the wonderful, amazing, life-changing technologies available to us today. We are in a new stage of existence, learning how to manage the never-ending opportunities to engage with each other and all the information we have to share. Perhaps technology itself will present a solution. We don't know. In the meantime, perhaps you could look out for little moments of nothing in your everyday life and see if you can't settle into them for a little while, indulge in a little 'stopping' before looking for a way out (reaching for your phone).

Maybe you'll find yourself sitting and gazing out the window a little more, staring into space while waiting for the kettle to boil, having a daydream when waiting for the bus. If your thoughts seem loud and irritating, just remember that it's simply your brain doing everything it needs to do before it can relax into its holiday (it's effectively checking the weather, booking the flights, picking out some new clothes. . .). Once it's done everything it wants to do (and you don't have to do anything to make sure that it does, apart from nothing), your brain will take its holiday, and, without you having done anything, your brain will be in an identical state to that of someone in meditation.

Whether you declare yourself a practitioner of meditation or mindfulness or not, your mind has a great capacity for emptiness that naturally arises when you do nothing. It is deeply comforting to reflect on the simple fact that we can't 'meditate' as an activity.

— Meditation happens to us all, very naturally, if we allow ourselves the simple act of doing nothing.

You have an exquisite meditation practice, and there's no reason for you not to do it in a café while your friend responds to a call of nature.

Rest is not only something you need no particular conditions, skills or knowledge to 'do' but it also has exponential value across the rest of your life. Stopping is not self-indulgent, it is not lazy, it is not a cop-out, and it is absolutely not a waste of time. On the contrary, when we allow ourselves to do nothing and just be, we start to experience the always-OK part of our experience. Our consciousness starts to shine forth through the gaps of our however-chaotic-or-not life, and we begin to feel the truth of the possibility that our essential nature is already rested and whole.

We might face a whole load of uncomfortable feelings, emotions and thoughts en route, but behind the boredom, the restlessness and the nagging feeling that we should be *doing something* to be better than we already are, we uncover a contentment that can be found in nothing and nowhere else but ourselves.

— *Our most contented self is already and always here.*

Enquiry 6:
What happens between breaths?

In *Enquiry 5: How are you breathing?* (see page 75) you most likely saw how your out-breath becomes longer as you rest. Now we can undertake some interesting enquiries by simply watching this exhalation more closely, and we want to pay particular attention to what happens at the *end* of the out-breath, namely the 'turn' in the breath – the moment when the exhalation switches to an inhalation.

If we keep watching, in time we might notice a moment of pause or sense some kind of 'space' that appears at the end of the exhalation. Importantly, this isn't something you should set out to create, as the effort will likely cause tension, reduce the exhalation and therefore be counter-productive.

As ever, your task is only to watch and let your body unfold its own relaxation response. This will bring you into a doubly powerful position: by observing the breath you will shift from thinking and move toward feeling/sensation (as in Enquiry 3, see page 46). It will help slow the breath, and then, by observing the exhalation, you will begin to naturally influence the length of this breath and create a further relaxation response in the body.

By 'doing nothing' you enter a self-supporting loop of ease following ease.

Your mind will likely wander from time to time. Let it. The more you try to force your mind to pay attention, the more tension you create. Be patient with yourself. This will be an imperfect experiment. All you can do is watch.

- *Prepare to rest (lie down, sit up, lounge in an easy chair, swing in a hammock – however you might feel most at ease)*

- *Begin to observe your breath. Just be with the breath for a little while, however you are breathing. Remember not to influence your breath*

- *Next, turn your attention, gently, to the moment when your exhalation transitions to the next inhalation*

- *Watch this moment for a few rounds of inhalation and exhalation*

- *Can you notice the feeling of this 'turn' in the breath? What is it like? Does the breath feel like it comes and goes, or is it more like a cycle? A wave?*

- *Watch the movement of the breath some more, and continue to notice how this transition feels*

- *As you pay attention to this experience of the breath turning, see if you can notice if there is any space between the movement. Is there a point at which everything stops? A moment in which you are neither breathing in, nor out?*

- *Keep with this possibility for a few breaths. Feel into it*

- Stay with this observation for as long as feels comfortable

- When you're ready to finish, allow your attention to return to the breath rather than the transitions, and pay attention to the feeling of breathing in

- Begin to move your body gently and bring yourself out of rest

Rest and Happiness

Most of us are motivated by the desire to be happy. A great deal of what we do and decide is informed by our intention to makes ourselves happier than we perceive ourselves to be right now. We identify particular objects, people, situations and places that we believe will bring us happiness, and we set out to get them. We often ignore or 'stuff down' emotions that we determine are in conflict with our potential to be happy.

We make happiness the end goal, and some of us will not rest until we achieve it.

But what is the payoff for this quest? Could it be possible that happiness is not dependent on anything at all? Could it be that happiness can come even when we have *done nothing* to make ourselves happy?

— Does getting everything we want really make us happy?

We've all heard of rich and famous people who have struggled with depression and yet we continue to imagine that if we had their wealth, we would be happy. We so easily forget that wealth is a complicated thing, with its own particular challenges and gifts, and we can say the same for poverty. There are people who claim that it was during times of lack that they felt most alive and most authentic, but to deliberately seek out a minimalistic lifestyle with the expectation that it will bring happiness might be just another way of defining yourself and your happiness by your wealth and possessions.

Most of us continue to run with the simple equation: money = happiness; poverty = suffering. Of course, when we're really struggling to make ends meet, more income and having enough food on the table will bring immediate relief, so perhaps more subtly, we confuse wealth with abundance. We think that after our needs are met the impact of having *more* in our life will continue to bring us relief and a feeling of security. We imagine we will feel satisfied and safe, when in fact we will most likely still have desires and fears – and these might even be amplified.

We can all think of that special something, someone or experience that brought something amazing to the surface of our life. We think about the item, the person or the event, and we are pleased by the thought.

But is there anything you could acquire that would improve that *underlying* feeling of ease and wholeness that presents itself to you when you are at rest – when you are only being? If you can remember the last time you were met by that sense of one-ness, of absolute silence and stillness, can you imagine there being anybody or anything that could fill you up *more* than your own sense of being? Could anything add more to that experience?

— When at rest, we need for absolutely nothing. There is no one thing and no one person capable of ever making us any more complete than we already are.

The point is, having nothing more than your basic needs met can be freeing, and having anything you want can also be freeing, but ultimately, they are two sides of the same coin and can be equally weighty traps or freedoms. We won't know how we will feel until we are in it, but we do know that neither one is going to leave us feeling any more complete than we feel when resting in our awareness.

Remember, awareness is necessarily spacious (it is aware of everything, right out to the stars and beyond) and impervious to material goods. Your *being* is always being, regardless of what it has or doesn't have. As we remember this, we feel full again – and how amazing to feel full from nothing!

Sometimes this remembering is fleeting, sometimes more sustained, but it is always a delight. Even if you do find yourself back on the high street or scouring the internet for that little something to give you a lift, you might now be less invested in the outcome of your pursuit. You might even find yourself enjoying the process more, knowing that you don't *need* it. There's already more joy in your pot – not because you set out to acquire joy, but because you know that regardless of what you have or want on the surface of your experience, the backdrop to all your experiences is an awareness that is entirely and always satisfied.

The deep quietness that you are able to feel when you stop is something that cannot be improved or eroded. The unshatterable is right here, right now within you, always. Whenever you touch back in to this feeling of being, you experience yourself as already whole, and nothing – no thing – can make you any better.

To embrace the possibility that happiness is not dependent on any particular thing does not mean you have to give up enjoying your possessions or taking on work that enables you to buy them. On the contrary, if you can embrace and love all of the stuff without seeing it as something that has the potential to complete you, then you're in with a chance of finding some peace and ease and a way to live that feels nourishing and entirely yours.

Some traditions advocate the absence of desire to be the only route to happiness. In real life, we tend to think the absence of desire, and therefore happiness, will only come once we have everything we want. But we can take a step back from both of these beliefs and see that we can have and fulfil desires on one level, while knowing that at our essence we are satisfied. We need not change how we live, but only how we define our lives.

When we are resting, we are wanting for nothing. We experience our being as completely satisfied, regardless of our hopes, plans, wish lists or goals. The fact that we have these desires though does not negate our inherent completeness at all.

ASK YOURSELF

Can you describe exactly what happiness is, or what has made you 'happy' in the past?

What do you really need?

We have to acknowledge that you, the reader, most likely have your basic needs met. You are likely to have shelter and enough food and water to survive. You might have a whole lot more than that, and good for you, but then there is also a chance that despite this, you still feel as though you don't have enough – that your life somehow needs *more*.

This feeling is nothing to be ashamed of.

Some people assume that to lead an awakened life you must renounce material possessions and show no interest in wealth, but again, this is putting conditions on the unconditional. For us, while financial gain is not our first priority when it comes to our work, we can admit we take satisfaction and pleasure in finding ways to share what we teach and earn a living from it. Sometimes, we like to treat ourselves. We find it pleasing to occasionally buy clothes that are not essential and enjoy being able to open the kitchen cupboard and be met with a luxury chocolate bar that, although our body doesn't need it, serves to bring as a few moments joy – in the anticipation of eating it, and then in the act itself. We even have a half-decent car that is fun to drive, comfortable on a long journey and was a bit flash in its day. These things – and more – bring us snapshots of pleasure, rushes of excitement and moments of enjoyable anticipation. They are small and largely inconsequential, but we like them nonetheless for it.

We are not ashamed to garnish our everyday life in this way and we are incredibly grateful to be able to do this while doing work that we love. Things haven't always been this way, and they might not be in the future.

Like most people, our default setting is that however much we have, we always want more. There's always a desire to *get* – get better, get bigger, get more. But this desire is not in itself a 'bad' thing, because it helps keep us motivated to work, create, grow, develop, chase our dreams and seek out new adventures. It is therefore a matter of maintaining perspective on the limits that material gains and prestige have in bringing us happiness, while remaining enthusiastic about where our talents and explorations might take us. We can enjoy the trappings of wealth and thrill of success without relying on them to define who we are or determine our value.

And we must remind ourselves that *things* are not the key to happiness. They have very little to do with our overall sense of being OK with who we are and what we are doing with our lives right now. It is a great privilege to be able to buy more than we need, but it is ultimately a short-lived pleasure and rarely felt very deeply. We try to remind ourselves and each other to be watchful whenever we seem to be chasing after *more* or seeking out opportunities that offer little other than financial gain. We try to be careful to not become slaves to our desire to have more than we need to feel OK.

Rest and the feeling that something is missing

Many of us feel as though there is a void within us that we must fill. 'Something's missing,' we bemoan, and we try to satisfy ourselves by adding more things, activities, experiences and people into our lives. It's a common theme for a lot of us, this feeling that we are missing out, or that we're lacking in something vital to our well-being, or that we are somehow being cut off from a rich and meaningful life. We look outside ourselves to see what might be missing – to correct the flaw, complete the puzzle, make ourselves feel full.

Feelings of lack might fuel our desires for something new or different or more, and these desires need not necessarily be ignored – to create, experiment, plot and imagine are the joys of being alive.

But what if this feeling of there being something missing comes back, regardless of how full we've made our lives? Could it be that this craving is us missing our own *being*? This familiar home ground of stillness?

When we rest, our desire to complete ourselves though acquisition and achievement tends to fall away. We are no longer looking outside ourselves; the simple experience of rest allows us to feel full and complete.

We might now even feel that unfillable space within us to be something of a sanctuary; a place in our experience that is free, uncluttered, unhindered and in need of nothing (because it *is* nothing).

If we can welcome this whole lot of nothing deep within our being, we might even feel liberated; we might see that at our essence, we are forever open and free.

ASK YOURSELF

How do you feel about your desires? Do you feel as though your happiness is dependent on them? Can you enjoy merely having the desire?

As we accept that we can always come back to this fullness (which is empty!) within us, we might feel lighter and less desperate to fill ourselves up with anything and everything we can. We might become more discerning in our choices. We might feel more at liberty to pick, choose and ponder, realising that after our basic needs are met, there is very little that can actually increase our overall sense of wellbeing. We might still want for more, but we also know that our wellbeing is not dependent on it.

Enquiry 7:
Can you find rest in the space between breaths?

If we turn our attention once again to the breath and that moment between the in-breath and the out-breath (see Enquiry 6, page 87) we have a window of opportunity to glimpse something of this stillness we've been talking about – this restful quality of our essential self.

When we exhale, we can observe all the way to the end of the breath until the breath changes direction. In this transition between breaths, you might notice the breath fading and building, much like watching waves break on the beach (if you performed the enquiry, then you might have your own description of this experience). If the body is becoming more naturally relaxed, there will be an 'outgoing tide'; that is to say, the breath going out will be a bigger wave than the breath coming in. It is worth noting again that we must not strive to manipulate a particular type of breath but observe how our breath just happens to be. We will most likely become absorbed in the process of watching the breath, which causes our bodies to relax and therefore engender a longer exhalation – it can only be effortless.

If you explored Enquiry 6 then you might have noticed how one breath dissolves into the next. There's a moment when the breath becomes unified, or we might say when the breath disappears into the one that's to come – the breath you were observing has fallen away and you're left waiting for the next. This moment between the end of the exhalation and the beginning of the next inhalation* – a pause before the turnaround – when you are neither inhaling nor exhaling, presents the opportunity to not only feel a space but also go deeper and notice what it's like to be aware of something (the breath) and then feel its absence.

In these moments, when the breath is gone and yet we remain there witnessing, we can ask ourselves who or what we are if we are neither breathing in nor breathing out. What is happening when nothing is happening?

Some say that this space – this happening of nothing – is what lies at the core of all yoga practices: to witness that which remains. To become aware of the space in which all objects appear (some call it 'subjective witnessing'). As you spend time in this space, rather than having another thought or idea about who you are, you are having a direct glimpse of the restful awareness that lies at the essence of your being.

Our minds love to objectify, and in this enquiry we have given the mind what it wants (we've let it follow an object – the breath in this instance) but then for a split-second the breath disappears and what's left behind is only the watchfulness.

This enquiry can be profoundly liberating or very confusing – and often it is both. The mind will try to objectify, again, and try to work out something that can't really be worked out. The mind will never be able to understand awareness because awareness is something beyond the mind. It is the space in which the mind appears. It is the part of our experience in which all our thoughts come and go. We cannot think it. We will never be able to work it out.

We have spent years interviewing our students to gather common language for this experience. While words will always fall short of something that the mind can't grasp, it is possible to describe how *resting* in that place between breaths impacts the body and mind. We can come back from this place and feel its residues in the body and mind. People have used all sorts of words to describe this experience, such as spaciousness, peace, restfulness, stillness, expansion, infinity, absorption and – a recent favourite – a 'tasty chaos'.

Although simple, this enquiry can be unsettling. You might find yourself getting lost in it and feeling spaced out afterwards. For many, it is a profound experience, though, of course, there will always be people who find it utterly uninteresting. This is life.

- *You can do this right now just as you are, or you can make a point of getting yourself comfy and away from distractions*

- *Close your eyes and watch your breath. Don't alter the breath. Just watch*

- *See if you can notice that pause – that space between the exhalation and inhalation. How would you describe it? How do you feel in that moment between breaths? What is happening in that moment?*

- Continue to observe your breath and explore (rest in, loiter in) that space – that moment between breaths – for a short while.

- See if you can sense how that moment between breaths becomes the background, and even as the next breath appears, feel how the moment that was just revealed lives on, like a backdrop to the breath

- Continue to be with that space. Fall back into it. See if you can even feel yourself *becoming* that space

- This is like a change of perspective: moving from being the breather, to being breathed, to *being* the space in which breath happens

- Remain with this spaciousness for a few moments

- When you feel ready to resurface, bring your attention back to your breath

- Move your body a little, and gently bring yourself back to wakefulness

* For some, the space at top of each breath (the end of the inhalation, before the exhalation) is just as good a place to explore as the space at the end of the breath – it might feel safer for you. It's really important that you do not *force* a gap between breaths. This is a surrendering practice; if you put any effort into it at all, it will elude you.

What do you want to feel?

Happiness is not a universally agreed feeling. When you think of happiness you might think of some kind of fizzy excitement or you might envisage a gentler sense of everything being OK. The question, 'Are you happy?' can point us towards a single particular sensation at a given time or it might lead us to enquire as to our general feeling over a longer period.

We might claim we want to be happy, but at the same time we know it is impossible to be happy all the time. Even if we were to be happy all the time, then it would become normal and probably wouldn't feel like happiness anymore. So, what do we want really?

There are countless books on the subject of how to be happy, and while, like anyone else, we enjoy those times in life when we feel at ease and are generally enjoying ourselves, we are also aware that difficult times are inevitable and, although it is hard to see it at the time, have their gifts, too. If we consider it properly, we don't really want to be happy *all* the time because we don't want to feel only one thing for the rest of our lives; we want to sample all aspects of life, and we want to recognise the importance of this especially during more challenging times.

If we constantly focus on happiness as the ultimate goal then we are danger of not being fully present with how things are in our lives right now. We might deem our current experience inadequate compared with an imagined experience in an imagined future. We give our present a demotion based on a future we do not know; we are not fully valuing the situation we are in.

We might have good reason for doing this, especially if we are faced with particularly testing times. To think that things are not going to improve might be too depressing a thought. The hope of a brighter tomorrow might be the only thing we can grasp on to to make the here and now feel bearable. It is a very difficult ask: to recognise that those things that bring you sadness, grief and pain are as valuable contributions to your existence as all of the 'good' stuff, and that you honour their appearance in your life.

— It's not all good, and that's good.

Bad ideas, bad feelings, bad thoughts, bad habits – they're as much part of your experience as all the so-called good stuff. They contribute to you being and feeling whole, or 'complete', or, our favourite: *balanced*. As we've already suggested, sometimes our bad experiences do more to leave us feeling at peace than the good. We learn, grow and blossom as a result.

That's not to say you should 'smile through' the hard times; quite the opposite, if you don't feel like smiling, you absolutely should not smile. There is a monumental difference between being accepting of your situation and forcing it into a positive framework. The former allows the 'bad' experience to present itself just as it is, without conditions on it changing or leaving. The latter is concerned with somehow finding a way to make that experience seem better (we might give it a story, or attach meaning to it that pleases us but may not be related to why it actually came into our experience). Whether you're putting on a brave face through grief or attempting to be friendly with a colleague you can't see eye-to-eye with, any attempts to 'be positive' come with the potential to be inauthentic and for the truth of the situation to not be given the attention it needs.

We're all for looking for ways to instantly feel a bit perkier, but the danger is that it can be ultimately quite destructive to shun your dark side – to turn your back on the nasty, uncomfortable and sometimes terrifying stuff that lies deep (or maybe not so deep) within yourself. Sometimes we need to feel sad. Sometimes we need to feel angry. Sometimes we need to recognise that we absolutely do not feel any gratitude whatsoever. These feelings are all part of who we are. To resist them and attempt to expel them from our experience is an act of self-denial.

We rarely *just listen* to ourselves, in the same way that we very rarely listen to anyone without agenda. We listen as though we were a committee working to find a solution. You might have had such an experience when sharing something difficult you're going through with a friend. Have you ever had that feeling that they have not so much heard you but merely sought to fix everything for you? It's a frustrating thing when all we want is to share how we're feeling – for our experience to be understood or validated – and instead we find our situation being boxed up with a neat little solution and packaged back to us ready for its disposal. We know that friend meant well, but all we really wanted was to bring our feelings to the surface and for it to be OK for them to be there.

We've all been that fix-it friend, and we've all been that friend in need, but we are very often both when it comes to listening to our own feelings. In our quest to be happy, we resist or even reject the more unpleasant 'messages' that arise from deep within ourselves, be they emotions, desires, memories, fears or physical sensations. Our immediate response is to try to send them on their way, either by presenting a solution or ignoring them. Perhaps, if we could imagine these 'unpleasant' sensations as friends visiting us then we will better see the value of just *being there* for them. We can listen without the intention or obligation to 'do' anything about what we hear.

Perhaps just considering this scenario offers you relief.

ASK YOURSELF

Can you simply acknowledge something you are grappling with right now without wanting to find a solution for it? Imagine yourself not trying to fix, push away or even understand an unpleasant situation or experience as it presents itself to you, and instead simply be with it, and ask if it wishes to share anything with you. The tension around the unpleasantness might diminish. . . without you having done anything.

Let's say you're aware of something dark beneath the surface – let's say it's a whisper of anxiety that rises to the top of your experience now and again, typically when you're feeling overwhelmed. The temptation might be to brush it under the carpet ('It's just an annoying little bit of nervous energy, after all, probably relating to [insert past event here that may or may not be related to present-day anxiety]'), but we're encouraging you to invite this feeling to present itself to you fully. We're suggesting you pull up a chair for it, make it a cup of tea, and listen to it.

The challenge is to resist the temptation to analyse the murkiest depths of your soul (as some therapies will have you doing) but more to create the space for the murkiest depths of your soul to present themselves to you, however they wish to do so, and for you to then discard any preconceptions about what they need, want or how they might leave.

We very often think we know what's going on inside, but all too often we've got the wrong end of the stick or distracted ourselves with a red herring or created a neat little story that we think explains/justifies all our woes. When we rest, when we have committed to do nothing and allow everything to present itself to us just as it wishes, the results (although we have not sought any) can be surprising. But we must be willing to only listen, otherwise, as soon as we start looking for answers and explanations, we've stopped really listening and we're back to creating a whole new bunch of stories and projections. Your innermost messengers are not going to stop communicating with you until you have uncon-ditionally received their communication.

We are not suggesting you spend the rest of your life sitting in a dark room having a party with your darkest thoughts, but if you can learn to stop approaching the uncomfortable aspects of your experience as though they are objects that must be turned into good aspects of your experience, then you will feel less burdened – less as though there is something that must be *done* about how you feel.

It is OK to just *feel*. It might be more important than you being happy right now.

Paradoxically, this always (certainly *nearly* always) leaves you feeling as though you have, without effort or agenda, found some peace with the issue at hand.

Enquiry 8:
Can you 'just listen'?

This enquiry asks you to explore what you may have previously considered 'noise' or distraction, and instead of ignoring or trying to 'block it out', listen.

Inevitably, the first thing that happens when we set about this enquiry is that you'll experience your mind to be like a table at a jumble sale – chaotic, random and full of junk. You might have the urge to rummage through and see if you can find something of value. However, while we might recognise this impulse, we're not going to act on it. We're just going to take time to observe what's on the table.

After a short while, something interesting might happen. You might begin to see themes, or recurring stories or feelings jumping out at you. At this point, you can enquire as to what seems to be calling for the most attention. What appears to be the *theme* of this jumble sale? You might notice a persistent thought or feeling, and you might see if there are any physical sensations relating to these themes. You might become aware of images running through your mind.

If a theme becomes apparent, see if you can welcome it in (your inclination might have been to ignore it, or mould into something more 'positive'). You can even actively engage with it and ask questions that might help you better discern what this visitor is asking of you.

This may appear to be a task-oriented enquiry, but remember, we are not intending to 'do' anything about the themes that appear, we are simply being present with them. We are looking at them, without agenda.

- Set yourself up for rest. Sit, lie down, stand, levitate if that's your thing. Apply what you already know about how you most easily access rest

- Close your eyes and start by only watching your thoughts. Don't worry about themes or stories yet, just watch and notice

- After a while, it may be that a theme emerges. It might be familiar to you – a regular or persistent visitor – or something quite unexpected or strange

- Firstly, notice how you feel about this 'guest'. How do you feel about it being here in your mind? How does it feel about you? Is there friendliness and accord, or is there refusal, denial or resistance from you or it?

- If there's a lack of harmony, your first move is to meet all of that resistance. How does it feel in your body? What's happens as you simply observe your relationship with this guest?

- As you get more familiar and comfortable with this visitor (this might take a few rounds of this enquiry) ask it if there is anything it's trying to show you

- As you ask this question, trust in the answers. They may at first seem abstract, strange or counterintuitive in some way. You don't need to take any action, but it's helpful to learn to trust your thoughts and perceptions. This might be the process of your unconscious mind revealing some new information to you – you can get to know your own process for insight

- Most importantly, don't try to figure anything out. This isn't an exercise in thinking or problem solving, but one of listening and allowing

- What else do you notice? Are there any images, changes to body sensations or other emerging feelings or emotions that might bring further insight?

- Spend as long as feels fruitful in this mode of listening. Take your time. Sometimes, your inner stories and characters might feel shy or untrusting of you. If you've been pushing something away for a while, it might take some time for you to change your relationship with this particular guest

- Finally, notice if there's some kind of action you might take that would help your guest feel seen and heard. What is needed for resolution? What would help it to settle down?

- If you get stuck in a loop of thinking – of trying to work things out – notice the sensations and feelings that accompany the narrative. Shift your attention from thinking about your thoughts to feeling them

- *When it feels right, see if you can acknowledge that feeling of 'being'; that there is something here that's aware of these inner themes that's not actually 'in' them. Exploring the space between breaths, as in Enquiry 6 (see page 87), can be a way to access that feeling of spaciousness and nothingness in which these thoughts are occurring*

- *After a short while of feeling this quality of spaciousness, begin to transition from your time of rest. Wiggle your fingers, move a little, and notice the sounds around you. Perhaps open your eyes and see the outer world, as a contrast to all that you've been seeing in your inner world*

Rest helps us to not be overwhelmed by our feelings

Anxiety is key contender for the most resisted and unwanted aspect of experience, and panic attacks in particular demonstrate how we get completely caught up in trying to find a solution to how we're feeling. When we feel panic arising within us, our heart starts to race and we start to feel physically unwell – perhaps even as though we are facing imminent death. Of course, we have an overwhelming desire to get rid of this feeling, because it's awful.

We look for a reason for this panic. We want to understand why it has come into our experience so that we can work out how we might be able to remove it. We might try various techniques to do this: focusing on a soothing thought, trying to slow our breathing. Very often, however, the racing heart and panicky feelings don't go away, and we start panicking even more about why they have come into our experience, what they mean and why they won't go away, and we continue with greater force to wish them away. We feel overcome by the panic and all our negative feelings about it. We resist the panic, and yet it remains, or even grows. We start panicking about the panic, and so it goes on. We feel as though we have *become* the panic. For this reason, anxiety tends to be an overriding and recurring gremlin in our life, popping up and spoiling our fun at the most unexpected and inappropriate of times.

So, what's the trick? Can we tell you how to get rid of this gremlin?

No.

Your anxiety has every right to make itself known to you whenever it so wishes. Your duty, as its host, is to allow it to be there, and to stop getting in its way and second-guessing its every move. When you next feel anxiety creeping in (because that's how anxiety tends to operate – she's a creepy fellow), imagine yourself taking her by the hand, sitting her down and asking her if she has anything she would like to talk about. Crucially: don't *force* her to tell you anything. If she just wants to sit there and be all creepy and quiet, so be it. The 'trick' is to remember that although you might prefer more amiable visitors, anxiety is just that – a visitor who comes and goes, and if she's being discourteous, so be it. Let her be. Don't take it personally. Get out of the way. If you resist her, she'll likely only fight back harder.

We cannot find happiness by ignoring our feelings

There is an enormous difference between letting things be and ignoring them. We might feel that turning a blind eye to things that we do not like or cannot be bothered with is one way to bring a sense of ease into our lives, but there is a risk that in doing so we are missing something important, either about ourselves or others, and there is the further risk that we cut ourselves off from our experience of life. We can remain steady amid turmoil because we have found an inner sense of ease, but we can also appear to remain steady amid turmoil because we have 'checked out'.

If you can embrace life not as an obstacle to be overcome or a future to work towards, but a perfectly impersonal happening of which you are present, you might resist the urge to edit how you feel about it. You might see that everything you are experiencing, feeling, sensing and even thinking right now is meant to be (and so it is), and everything that is happening between those 'happenings' – your constant awareness, your 'ultimate presence' – is unfazed.

But this does not mean you cannot have preferences or opinions. If we can consider that our wellbeing is not dependent on us only experiencing 'positive' feelings, events and people, then we might be more willing to engage with our present circumstances, listening to our heartfelt emotions and trusting in our responses to them. If you are outraged by something then you should explore that outrage (invite it in, ask it if it has anything it would like to share with you – there might be an interesting insight, a surprising action you feel compelled to take as a result).

A little while ago, we found ourselves getting quite worked up about an issue that we will loosely describe as 'political'. We got animated whenever discussing it with friends and took action by joining local groups and signing petitions and encouraging others to do so. On observing this, an acquaintance of ours became quite annoyed; not by what we were saying as such, but more because she thought we shouldn't be saying anything at all. How, as teachers who promote balance over extremeness, and acceptance over resistance can we be so vocal about wanting to effect a change?

Perhaps naively, it had never occurred to us that people might interpret our call to 'stop striving and start being' as a way of advocating a disengagement from life – that the call was regarding external events, not internal.

To feel at peace, you do not need to create peaceful circumstances. To feel balanced, you do not need to orchestrate a balanced life-style. To accept who you are and what is happening to you, you do not need to alter the comings and goings of your life.

There *is* a world out there, and it's very much yours to engage with in a way that is in accordance with your truth (no one else's). You can have a busy, creative, full and productive life, all the while feeling at ease with who you are, the challenges that present themselves and how you respond to them. This is the very point of rest – of stopping and being with who you are and to engage with the very truth of your experience and existence.

Through rest we can find clarity, insight and awareness. Rest may appear to involve a passive detachment from experience, but on the contrary, it is a vehicle to connect, completely, to the very essence of who you are. This essential self is not resting and it isn't not resting; it just is. We might be urging you to unplug from your distractions, but we are not suggesting you unplug from yourself.

— *By resting, we become better able to discern our true desires, passions and needs.*

When we allow ourselves to stop and rest, and as we stop resisting the seemingly non-stop murmurings of our mind, the more likely it is that our deeper thoughts and sensations will start to bubble to the surface. The white noise diminishes, the mist clears, the curtain lifts. We retain our personalities – indeed, we get to see ourselves more clearly – and we may well become more focused and driven. Rest can and often is a precursor to activity, and proper rest will engender action that is most connected with your truest self.

Stopping, listening, allowing and enquiring are all gentle exercises in being, though that doesn't mean the outcome will be gentle. Maybe you'll see that the relationship you've been plodding along in for years really must come to an end. Perhaps you'll recognise how your work is making you unhappy. Perhaps you'll see that you really do need to write that uncomfortable letter to your father. A life of rested awareness is not one that will be easy; though you will live your however-challenging-it-may-be-life with clarity and authenticity. You will be 'at ease' with yourself, despite life perhaps not being, on the surface, easy on you.

We can approach our lives not as a pursuit of self-improvement but self-realisation, and take relief from the knowledge that above and beyond it all, whether experiencing happiness, sadness, grief, frustration, delight, exhaustion or confusion, we are fundamentally harmonious and complete.

As we rest and stop and allow for a glimpse of the essence of ourselves beyond our thoughts, beliefs, sensations and emotion, we are recharged by the knowledge that we have everything we ever need for whatever life hurls into our experience. We are fully synched. We are eyes-wide open living this life in the way that only we were meant to. This realisation might bring you happiness, and many more things beside.

Rest and Control

Some of us are afraid to stop. We fear that we will lose control and everything will fall apart. We feel stressed at the thought of carrying on, but equally stressed at the thought of stopping. We believe it is down to us to ensure things are one way or another, and we put off 'relaxing' until we are sure we have done everything possible to ensure events are shaped the way we wish them to be.

Then, even if we do succeed in ensuring everything is just as we want, we might become even more afraid of stopping, because we've proven to ourselves that our constant input is what shapes things into the way we wish them to be. And so we feel we must continue shaping and controlling and planning, and so we don't stop, and we never relax, and we can't rest, and we never glimpse into that place at the depths of our being where everything is OK just as it is all the time regardless of our doings or not doings. We can't even imagine such a thing is there.

Hopefully we have already led you along a path of enquiry that has to some degree liberated you from the mercy of unpredictable events and emotions that can knock you out of balance and inhibit your willingness to engage with yourself and your life just as it is. Rest, we hope you are beginning to see, is both the outcome and pathway to stillness – a stillness that holds you in all experiences, always. When we rest, we are resting into ourselves – we are held by something greater than our thinking and feeling, beyond our control though completely, utterly *us*.

Your relationship with rest has a great deal to do with your desire for control: your desire to control how you feel, what you experience, and even what you think. When you are resting, you are controlling nothing. To rest fully, you must surrender, but this is not from a place of 'giving up'; more, it comes from trusting in what lies beyond your control.

However, this trust can seem hard to find. Whether we consider ourselves a 'control freak' or not, we all, to a lesser or greater degree, have a desire to control numerous aspects of our experience, from our feelings, thoughts and practical circumstances to the feelings, thoughts and behaviour of others. This desire for control is generally amplified the less 'happy' we feel about something. This is when our ability to rest appears diminished; we cannot let go and stop because we feel desperate to reorder everything into a way that we believe will make us feel better.

It is completely normal to be forever thinking about what we must be doing next while engaging ourselves in a constant narrative, mind-chatting away about subjects that are sometimes completely irrelevant to the here and now, all the while desperately trying to control our experience and influence our place within it. But some of us can get completely overwhelmed by the sense of responsibility that comes with believing the events of our life, and our responses to them, are entirely of our own making. Our inner narratives start to inhibit our ability to recognise and respond to the here and now, or they might even make us too afraid to engage with our current circumstances and emotions. We become unable to be present with the situation we are in because we are busy preparing for a different one.

Were our ancestors, when staring out over the planes of Africa, thinking their equivalent of, 'I really must email Charlie' or 'I forgot to put the bins out' or even, 'Ooh, I like that tree, the way the sunlight is casting that shadow. How can I capture it so I can look at it again sometime?'. Do we see birds and rabbits and cats and dogs entering such internal debates? It's unlikely; science remains divided as to whether animals have a sense of time and we're in no position to guess, but we're fairly confident they're not analysing their childhood upbringing or worrying about the success of tomorrow's presentation in the context of how it's going to make them look amid their peers.

Your internal narrative is not going to stop, and this is just as it should be. You will always have endless, constant and multiple narratives running through your mind most of the time. The freedom and the relief comes not from finding a way to stop them, but from being able to step back from them – to become less caught up in them (to become *less* them entirely).

So how can we take this step back even when things seem in desperate need of our input? How can we be 'at one' with life even when life feels tumultuous, or even as though it is conspiring against us? And how can rest help us to see that our experience of life is not entirely our responsibility?

How can doing nothing help us to feel less burdened by the desire to control our experience?

Rest: cause and effect

In times when we consider ourselves generally happy, we usually mean that on the whole things seem good with life. We're healthy, we're enjoying our work (or we're enjoying not working), and we are surrounded by people we love and who love us. We are not struggling.

If you have ever gone through such a period you probably didn't leap out of bed with a grin on your face every morning, skip to the bus stop and perform a dance number just because you were feeling so buzzed. You just felt at ease – life felt *balanced*. You were not in resistance to the events you were experiencing or the people around you. There was nothing you felt the urge to change. You might still have had desires and ambitions, but you probably weren't feeling overwhelmed by obligations or stressed by your to-do list.

These easier periods of life tend to come together for all number of reasons, some of which we might have worked hard to orchestrate, while others just sort of seem to happen by chance but that we feel are signposts that things were 'meant to be'. This is the beauty of these periods: we feel both blessed by the universe (or whatever we might believe has the power to align – or not – events with our hopes) and proud of ourselves. We feel a sense of unison. The downside is that just as these periods of 'everything's going my way' can enter our lives, they can also leave. Things start to come into our experience that we don't like (perhaps a relationship breakdown, or ill health, or even anxiety that we might attach to any one particular aspect of our experience). We go from being in a place we equated with 'ease' to a place of 'unease' (or even 'dis-ease') and disharmony. Suddenly, things are 'not good' and we proclaim ourselves 'not good' (and we might even start to feel bad about the fact that we don't feel good), and we embark on a quest to find the 'good times' again. We enter resistance with our life. We don't trust in the universe or God (or whatever higher power we might believe in) to align with our wishes. We wish to regain control.

We might also develop a kind of nostalgia for how we felt before life became difficult (we might recall a dance number at the bus stop).

There is a whole lot of uncomfortable thinking (and feeling) going on in such circumstances. While we can't 'think' away our thoughts (or our feelings), we can explore our perspective and see if we can experience a turnaround without denying or resisting any of our genuine feelings about our situation. We can acknowledge our desire for things to be different, without specifying conditions for how that might come about.

Let's consider the following phrases:

I will feel better about my life if I find a job I enjoy
I will feel better about my life if I lose 10kg
I will feel better about my life when I find a girlfriend

We're putting conditions on our feelings by declaring that a particular change in circumstances will bring about a specific emotion. We forget that a feeling of 'OK-ness' very often comes without conditions.

Now let's turn these phrases around:

When I feel better about my life, I will find a job I enjoy
When I feel better about my life, I will lose 10kg
When I feel better about my life, I will find a girlfriend

ASK YOURSELF

Is there any particular thing you are banking on to 'improve your life'? How do you feel if you change the terms of your expectation; i.e. 'If I feel better about my life, this desire will be met'?

The latter situations are not necessarily less likely than the former, and yet we rarely consider them as being as much of a possibility. Perhaps they are even more likely – how often have you heard of a friend finding their soul mate as soon as they gave up looking? Or a couple finding themselves expecting their first born just weeks after they accepted parenthood was after all not on the cards for them and gave up trying? We've all had either friends or relatives who've found their way just as they made peace with their current situations. It's happened to us.

We are not encouraging you try to instantly make yourself 'feel better' about your life (a near impossible task) but to consider, with more scrutiny, how you might be placing conditions on your feelings. You might be determining yourself completely in control of them, and aware of what causes you to feel a certain way, when, as we have explored, things are rarely so straightforward.

A turnaround in your feelings about an aspect of your experience can come not by 'positive thinking' (or 'shifting your vibration'), but by recognising that the stories you might be attaching to your experiences, and their related feelings, might not be true – that you are not as in control of any of it as you might think. You can recognise that you feel loneliness, for example, but that you don't know what this might mean in regards to your ability to be at ease with your life. If you can let go of all your stories about that loneliness and instead allow it to be there just as it is, although the uncomfortable feeling remains, with it now comes an acceptance. The loneliness is present, but the power and stories you previously gave to it as a means to shape your feelings about your life are diminished. You have not put a veneer on your situation or your feelings, you have not tried to re-frame them into something positive, you have simply allowed them to be just as they are.

And it's here that the magic often happens: the discomfort from the feeling lessens (perhaps even dissipates) and we find ourselves if not 'happy' then certainly OK. Without our circumstances having changed or even our feelings about the circumstances, we are more at ease. We can be both 'unhappy' about our circumstances, but we can be at ease with our unhappiness – less overwhelmed by it, less attached to it, less *it*. We discover a sense of OK-ness that is there regardless of what is happening to us.

This is a superpower that we can all harness if we'd only be more allowing of what *is*.

Finding relief in seeing that your thoughts are not who you are

When we rest, we experience ourselves as the awareness that exists beyond our stories and beyond the events of our lives. We see that this existence is complete and balanced. However, when we are not resting, the stories we run – the thoughts that we have – seem as though they *are* who we are.

To a certain extent we can follow trains of thought and redirect them and actively start thinking about one thing or another, or switch one thought out for another. We can think about something sad to stop the inappropriate giggles or put on a comedy programme when we're in need of lighter thoughts. We can stop ourselves having that extra doughnut (but not always. . .). We can have a negative thought about somebody, and then actively think about everything we do like about them to change, if only a little, how we feel about them. We can put our mind to a maths puzzle or crossword, form arguments, recall dates, plan journeys and create imaginary worlds and stories. We can direct our minds as a resource on a certain level, but at the same time we can never be totally confident of what's coming next or how we might find ourselves approaching a particular task.

A thought can pop up out of nowhere that seems remarkably off topic (or remarkably *on* topic). We know that no amount of consideration and contemplation right now can prepare us for the thoughts we might have in the future: while working through the year-end spread sheets you might be surprised by a childhood recollection, or suddenly remember something you must add to your shopping list, or be hit by guilt because you haven't telephoned your father for a couple of weeks, or be baffled by something you've never understood about ancient Rome, or catch a nostalgic whiff of something relating to an ex-partner, or recall the name of the film you've seen that actor in before. . . anything, *anything* is possible.

If you spend some time to be with this predicament, it can be unsettling. Who's in charge here? If your own thoughts can take you completely by surprise, then where are they coming from?

ASK YOURSELF

What are you thinking right now? What will you be thinking
in five minutes' time? Five seconds?

A neuroscientist might say your thoughts come from a cluster of
neural-synapses grouped together in the pre-frontal cortex; a philos-
opher might say they arise from your interactions with life and
your mind's past. Both might be true, but neither really answers
the question entirely. There's still a definite element of mystery,
and certainly a possibility that your thinking is not down to *you*.
There is an interesting, and if you allow it, liberating lack of
responsibility here. Perhaps your thoughts are not *yours*.

Everything you believe comprises who you are – your thoughts
and beliefs and the emotions, feelings and sensations that accompany them – are not necessarily yours, in that they are a reaction
to countless happenings that were mostly not of your choosing
and largely out of your control. From the very beginning, life
happened to you. It's a clichéd and much-ridiculed comeback from
teenagers to shout, 'I didn't ask to be born!' but they do have a
point. They had no decision at all in their coming into this world,
and then so much more. From how their parents looked after and
loved them, to where they lived and what they ate and where they
went to school and who became their friends; it was utterly out
of their control.

This all goes against the popular belief that we can lead the life we choose, but the fact is so much of life happens *to* us. We do not make most of it happen. In some ways, it is not so much that we are living *our* life, but that life is happening around us. We are amidst multiple happenings.

In the same way, we tend to take a very personal perspective when it comes to all our 'stuff' – our 'emotional baggage'. Not only do we wholly and fully identify with our thoughts about our life but we also believe those thoughts to be ours and that the way we think and behave is entirely of our own doing. We berate ourselves for our behaviour or our inability to resolve situations and break so-called bad habits. We might enter cycles of 'inappropriate behaviour' followed by shame or various fix-it endeavours, which fail, and then comes the shame again. Whether it's how we eat, how we exercise, how we enter relationships, how we approach our careers, so many of us feel bad about who we think we are and the life we seem to be creating for ourselves. We see ourselves as failures, or that we are the only ones who didn't get the 'life handbook' or that we have substandard minds – that we are broken, or worse, that we broke ourselves.

ASK YOURSELF

Have you made an effort to change your behaviour, and then 'failed'? If so, how did you feel about that?

We don't all have these battles, but if you do, you might want to consider stepping back from your responsibilities here (again, perhaps not a very popular suggestion) and reflect on the possibility that so much of who you consider yourself to be is the result of things that have happened *to* you as opposed to you having made them happen. Countless and endless occurrences outside your control have crafted you into this unique and quirky being that you are today, so recognise that although you may be navigating a bumpy path, the bumps are not 'yours'. You are on a journey; the terrain is not you, and it is not your job to fix the terrain and nor is there any reason to assume that because the terrain is bumpy you are any less of a person on any less of a journey.

Knowing that so much of your thinking and responses to situations are as they are for reasons outside of your control can soften the self-criticising, self-judging voice. If we can recognise that what we take so personally is very much *impersonal*, then we might not only feel less of a sense of shame about what we do, think and feel, but also be less afraid to listen to ourselves, and let others see who we really are.

If you've ever felt ashamed or even just a little self-conscious about yourself or something you have done (or not been able to do), then you will know how strong the urge can be to hide. When we feel shame we are often also grappling with fears around rejection: just as we wish to reject aspects of who we are and what we have done, we edit ourselves in an attempt to present the version of us we think people wish us to be (so that they do not reject us). This inevitably leaves us feeling even more ashamed of who we are, and inauthentic to top it off. And so the cycle goes on. Our attempts to control who we are leave us feeling very much unlike ourselves, and we set about yet another regime to 'sort ourselves out' or we might even take measures to 'go find ourselves', which so often involves great expense and extensive travel yet so rarely involves the one thing we do need to find ourselves: to go nowhere and do absolutely nothing.

As ever, we wish to offer a counterbalance to this assertion. To qualify everything we have shared with you about the possibility that your thoughts and your experience of life are not personal, we must also assert the possibility that this does not make you a victim. Just as we urge you to step away from your beliefs that you are responsible for who you are and how you feel about your life right now, we must also urge you to step away from the opposite: that you are who you are entirely as a result of other people's actions against you. Remember, we are all navigating these bumpy paths, and at times, paths will inevitably cross.

— Life does not conspire against any of us, it just is.

Just as many of us feel responsible for what we believe are our failings, many of us feel as though we are being made to fail. Perhaps we blame our upbringing or the society in which we live, or maybe even a particular person who we feel has somehow 'ruined' us. Again, these beliefs although not 'wrong', because we are all who we are as a result of infinite happenings, can only ever be inaccurate – an assumption, a deduction, a summation. Such thoughts are never fact, and so while you must honour them, you can also respectfully take a step back and find that place in the middle: where you recognise you are neither in control of nor being controlled by life. There is no control.

Enquiry 9:
Can you give up control?

This is a simple enquiry around one thing: control. During the process, you take a mental 'posture of consciousness', which means that you simply allow every experience to be. Whether it is something that feels good or bad, it is welcomed equally. There is no choosing or refusing, no changing or holding on.

Whether it's a feeling, emotion, thought, sound or disruption. . . it's all allowed. We're asking you to let go of the need to control any aspect of your experience in any way. This requires your complete commitment, and bravery (for just a short while).

- *Prepare yourself for a few moments of doing nothing. It doesn't matter whether you sit or stand. You can have your eyes open or closed*

- *Now, for this entire time (however long you've chosen to perform this enquiry), surrender fully to your experience. Don't try to change a SINGLE thing*

- *Not. A. Thing*

- *See what happens. Do you feel at ease with surrendering control? Does it make you tense? Frightened? Agitated? Relaxed?*

- *This could be a very telling experiment for you*

- *Notice how there might be a quality participating in this experiment that is already utterly surrendered*

- *If 'you' can't surrender, what part of you is aware of this? Can you sense if there is an aspect of your awareness that might already be surrendered? Or that doesn't care whether you surrender or not?*

- *Don't try to pin down this part of your experience. Recognise it as always and forever here, and let all of your control (or the lack of it) rest in that possibility*

- *Keep allowing and being with everything just as it is for as long as you are able*

- *When you are ready, move your body, observe a few rounds of your breath, and resurface*

Remembering our being

It's all very well to recognise the limits of our control, but sometimes our experience of life means we feel we have a good idea of how things are going to turn out. We can see this at the most basic level: we know that if we open the fridge, we'll sense the cold air within it. If we turn the ignition, the car will probably start (not always, of course). We do know that certain causes and certain effects are largely inevitable. Our proposition is this: not that you know nothing, but that you know far less than you think you do. You are not always right, and very often your plans either don't turn out the way you had intended or your plans, even if expertly executed, don't have the effect you had imagined.

Sometimes, you make no plans and amazing things happen. Life is constantly surprising, even if in the most mundane of ways.

As we've already illustrated, you don't know what you will be thinking at any point in the future, and in this way you can appreciate that thoughts are arbitrary. Therefore, on the one hand we have knowledge, the bank of our experience, observations and our ability to problem solve, interpret and predict, and on the other we have our thoughts – how knowledge presents itself to us – and which are fickle, random and sometimes completely irrational. Coupled with this is that despite our knowledge, events can always unfold unexpectedly (the fridge may be broken, the car battery flat).

ASK YOURSELF

Can you recall an event that unfolded in a way you had not imagined it would? How did you feel afterwards?

Regardless of everything we know, we are taken by surprise more often than we might imagine. We are only ever hedging our bets and taking a guess. We do so fervently and passionately in the belief that it is more than a guess, but all the while there is part of us completely open and present with everything as it just so happens to be – never surprised or disappointed at the outcome of anything.

This awareness we've been pointing you towards (helping you to remember, to glimpse, to catch just a moment of), this exquisite feeling of inner stillness that exists behind all of the doing and knowing and having, is something that naturally comes and goes out of our experience. It's not something you can do or become good at. We don't know anyone who is always *being*.

Rest offers a window for us to dive into that place of being, but we very rarely remember this opportunity is there. This is because it is such a hard concept for the mind to grasp. Indeed, your mind will never be able to grasp it. It is beyond acquisition, past the thinking mind and not a thing to be found. Furthermore, it never leaves us, so we never notice its absence (try to think about that. . .).

Life, in all its busy, elaborate intricacy, naturally pulls us toward being *in* our experiences rather than *being* in the experiencing. We live as though there is not something essential within us impervious to all the comings and goings of life. We lose sight of our inner stillness because of its very nature.

The good news is that although we can't go looking for it (it's always here), and we certainly can't engineer it, we can take immediate relief in *remembering* our essential nature. We forget, get busy, get lost in the stuff of life and then we can remember that there's something else here too that's unchanging, still, unwavering and deeply restful. Just as on a cloudy day we forget that the blue sky remains behind, your mind forgets that regardless of what it's doing, your inner stillness is always there.

In this way, we can approach rest as if it were a game of hide and seek: as we settle down to sleep or take a nap or sit for meditation (or just sit and be, without having to give it a name), we can do so not so much with the intention of catching a glimpse of our essential self but as a response to the glimpses we have caught in the past and what they revealed to us.

By approaching rest in this way – by removing the need for rest to look one way or another – we have placated the mind's need to seek an outcome and allowed ourselves the opportunity to see beyond our thinking mind. We rest in the remembrance of having seen behind the curtain and caught sight of our essence – that which sits beyond control. We are not resting in order to catch a glimpse, but because we remember that our past glimpses came about when we rested.

In time, as we continue to make time to be – or be more – in the times we already have, such as watching our children play, or noticing the birdsong as we set about our daily commute, these micro-remembrances and glimpses add to our experience of being, and our sense of our inner stillness grows more familiar. There can be moments now in life when we're conscious of a pause even amid the hurrying pace of life. We're able to be for a moment, and it acts like a reset. Without effort or objective, we find ourselves building a bank of these snapshots, and so the remembering becomes easier, the glimpses of this 'stillness' more familiar and the mind less resistant to them. We find it easier to fill ourselves up with those moments of emptiness, which make life feel all the more full.

Ultimately, the stillness begins to come *to* us, and we experience it as integral to life. We become more able to feel our *being* amid our doing. We are controlling our lives perhaps no less, but we are stepping back from the outcomes of that control. It is not that we have any more of anything within us, we are merely more aware of that which was there all along. The quandary, as ever, is that we cannot enter rest with the intention of any of this happening; the future and any intentions for the future must be abandoned.

— *We are doing no less, but we are being more.*

Control and conflict

It is difficult to let anything go — to abandon our beliefs, hopes and hang-ups — and this is felt particularly strongly when we hope to influence another person's beliefs about how they see us or how they see a particular situation. This urge to influence another's thinking can leave us feeling desperately unsettled. We feel we need to make others see the way we see, and we want them to see that we are right.

When we enter arguments with our friends, family, co-workers or whoever, it's very easy to turn things into a war of understanding. Typically, both sides determine that they have the absolute facts and correct interpretation of those facts. Rarely does either party consider the actual fact: that neither has complete clarity of the situation. That's the challenge with knowledge: unless it's non-subjective truth (and there isn't much of that regarding us humans, as we always have angles/biases/various lenses through which we filter experience), it's limited. Why are we so unwilling to acknowledge this?

There are many answers to that question (we could discuss the concept of the ego, of survival, of competition. . .) but instead let's use it as an opportunity to find an easier way to be.

If we can consider that those with whom we have conflict, including ourselves, do not have all the facts about the issue or situation to hand, then we are receptive to the possibility that there might not need to be a resolution, or that the resolution will come in a way we had not expected. If we relinquish the need to know, and the need to make other people see what we know, then resolution must come from elsewhere. Perhaps our feelings about the issue will shift, or perhaps they won't and, somehow, we just won't care as much that they are not acknowledged to be 'true' by someone else, because we know there is no such thing as true knowledge. Our need to change, analyse and influence both ourselves and others, softens. The walls are removed, and there is greater possibility for insight.

ASK YOURSELF

After an argument, have you ever found that the resolution came, in effect, 'out of nowhere' or at least, from somewhere unexpected?

— *When we worry less about demonstrating what we know and proving our theories to be right, we're better able to just show up and listen.*

We can allow whatever comes in to the room to be fully seen and heard, whether it's the argument of a friend or our own inner conflicts. We can give it space: space in the room and the spaciousness of our own wholeness and OK-ness.

This is an incredibly potent approach to dealing with anyone, whether it's a friend in need, an enemy on the rampage or a person merely coming to you with information. When we listen, without wanting to know it all or demonstrate that we already know it all, there is far greater opportunity for profound insight and resolution.

How can we live knowing that we cannot know it all?

We live amid the unknowable, and the choice we have is to either strive to know (which we can never do) or *rest in not knowing*. Our intellect is necessarily limited, outcomes are ultimately unknowable, some thoughts just happen. With this we are off the hook. We cannot ever know. We cannot ever control. We are never entirely responsible.

As co-authors of this book, partners in 'real life' and parents to two children, we have many moments when one of us needs help to remember this. Typically, trouble brews when one of us has becomes contracted around a certain set of thoughts and beliefs, fearing the worst, and obsessing over the perceived likely negative outcome.

The temptation might be for one to assure the other that 'everything will be OK', and while this might be the case, it can never be known until after the fact. Therefore, instead, we offer each other the service of helping the other to *remember to forget*. When one of us gets lost in second-guessing the future or making up events out of how things are right now, the other can reflect this back to them – reminding them that they do not know how anything will be in the future. At first, being reminded of this can be painful, our little self becomes defensive – that part of us that wants to be right, even if it's about something going terribly wrong. Over time, as we are reminded more, and remind ourselves, it becomes easier to let go of the thoughts that bind us (and sometimes torment us) and we can more readily rest in not knowing. When you are able take a step back and see your thoughts about the future for what they are – supposition – it's like taking a deep bath. You might feel it in your body – a release perhaps, as you free yourself from that which you cannot know.

Enquiry 10:
What is it like to 'rest in not knowing'?

In this enquiry, we get a little more familiar with letting go of control and take relief from the realisation that we cannot know and, therefore, cannot be responsible for everything – and indeed far less than we could ever dare imagine.

Generally, we want to work stuff out. We want to have answers, solve the problem, get it sorted. We spend a lot of our lives analysing the apparent facts, weighing up pros and cons, and making choices and plans accordingly. This is one of the great tasks of the thinking mind – to help keep us safe, ahead of the game and on track with our ambitions. However, whereas this is all very helpful *in* life, it's not something that helps us when it comes to resting. Our most rested, essential self is way beyond our thinking mind and not something we can ever 'figure out'.

We can give our brains a holiday by allowing them to chatter away without any pressure to find the answers. Any questions that come up can simply be left unanswered. Any quandaries, propositions, ideas or realisations can be noticed, and then left alone. Everything is allowed to be there, and leave of its own accord (if it wishes).

In this enquiry, we rest into the feeling of letting go of the need to know anything at all. We wallow in the joy of our essential nature not needing us to figure anything out. We loiter in that part of our being – the space – that holds all the answers, whether they're 'right' or 'wrong' or somewhere in between.

The enquiry reminds us that we don't need to know it all – that we cannot ever know it all – and that this makes us no less complete.

- *Prepare for rest, however you wish – lying, sitting, indulging in an adolescent slouch*

- *Close your eyes. Accept that your thinking mind will not at once buy into this 'brain holiday' and that thoughts will come and go*

- *You'll most likely notice a lot of thoughts*

- *Even more thoughts*

- *Instead of thinking about not thinking (you will!), see if you can allow your thoughts to come and go, however they wish*

- *See if you can relinquish your interest in your thoughts. See if you can allow them to become background noise, like listening to static or a detuned radio*

- *If you do want to engage in a thought, make it one about the concept that right now, there is nothing you need to know*

- *See if this thought can dissolve into more of a contemplation, and then a feeling*

- *See if you can let go of any concepts, certainties and outcomes that your mind will surely produce in regard to this contemplation*

- Remember that there's nothing that you need to know in order to rest. Rest is already here, behind all concepts

- Continue to rest, and let go of any need to produce answers

- If a thought comes, you can't pretend it isn't there, but you don't have to 'answer' it

- Continue with this for a few minutes (or many minutes, if you have time)

- When the time feels right (if indeed you are aware of time), move your body a little, take a breath, and resurface

Rest and resolution

When we allow whatever feelings, emotions, thoughts or images that wish to present themselves to us to be heard, there may well be a number of outcomes. The tricky thing is that the very desire to have an outcome might hamper your ability to truly listen.

(You see how you must let go, and then let go of letting go. . ?)

The first outcome, and this may at first seem disappointing, might be that there is *no* outcome. By simply paying attention and welcoming, we have begun the process of establishing an inner harmony. We have begun listening to ourselves and trusting ourselves, even though the situation or experience might still feel quite unresolved (the anxiety might still be there, but we have taken a step back from it, and feel less like we *are* it). This in itself brings around a sense of equilibrium, and certainly a sense of authenticity.

A deeper potential outcome is that having listened and welcomed, the feeling or thought begins to soften, open and bubble up to the surface. Perhaps nothing has been resolved practically or outwardly, but the inner world begins to let go of the resistance and we find out that the 'problem', although still there, is less of a disturbance.

A deeper outcome further still might be that we receive an insight from our subconscious, perhaps in the form of an image, some words or a shift in sensation. As we enter into communication with ourselves and are listening and even, with practice, *trusting* that we are capable of resolving our own conflicts without *doing* anything about them, our inner world presents some new information for us. This information might not be convenient: it might be the insight that we need to have an uncomfortable conversation with somebody or take an action that goes against our traditional response to a situation. This is growth, however daunting or painful, and it enables us to work towards a new pathway of interacting with the world. At least, that might be the way of describing this development if we were to intellectualise it. The underlying feeling, though, is one of things seeming that they are as they should be – just as when our intuition *knows* something is the right thing to do or say (or *not* do or say) even if our 'thinking mind' is in resistance.

How can I be restful towards overwhelming emotions?

There are times when aspects of our experience – a memory, a shocking incident, grief – are overwhelming, and taking a step back is seemingly impossible. We cannot see ourselves as the host to this particular 'visitor,' or perhaps we can, and the visitor turns out to be a maniac who simply won't leave.

Furthermore, as we listen to one 'visitor', we might receive a message or insight that is perhaps even more unpleasant than its messenger, and so we might have another layer of 'unpleasantness' to welcome. To be able to receive these messages without our brains diving in and trying to make everything better can take some courage (and in some circumstances, when we start to feel unsafe, we should ask someone who understands the process to be with us as we do so).

Sometimes, regardless of how much we have 'listened', we continue to feel stuck with the negative feelings that arise within us, so what particular flavour of 'nothing' must we do in such a situation?

The first thing is to say that it might be wholly necessary for us to *be* stuck for a while. If you rush to get away from the experience of feeling stuck, then you're back into the running-away loop of experience and avoiding your feelings. So, in the first instance, see if you can allow the stuckness to be there. Explore how that feels. Treat the stuckness as another visitor. Offer it the proverbial cup of tea.

ASK YOURSELF

Is there anything in your life (a recurring feeling or a habit, maybe) that you feel you just cannot move on from? Can you allow that feeling of being stuck with it to be present in your experience for a while? Can you relax the desire to become unstuck?

If this feels unsafe for you, if you continue to feel overwhelmed by the experience, a well-timed question could be just the very thing to shift your perspective. We are not going to ask anything to leave, but more offer a cushion for it to sit on. Let's take the example of a person in pain, an experience that in addition to the physical often leads to extreme and understandable mental discomfort. When pain is present, it's hard to imagine it ever leaving, and indeed, this is very often the fear. However, making ourselves answer a question relating to this fear can enable us to see the other possibility:

'Is it true that the pain will never go away?'

We are not fortune-tellers, so we do not know whether the pain will go away or not. The answer can only be, 'No'.

We can then consider how contemplating the possibility of it leaving makes us feel.

'How do I feel when I consider the pain might go away?'

'Can I describe how it would feel to not be in pain anymore?'

By answering such questions, focusing on our feelings (perhaps noting any physical sensations in the body, even when we are not exploring physical pain), we can subtly shift out of one particular groove and gently feel into the possibility of another outcome. We now have in our experience the pain as well as the possibility of the absence of pain. We are neither denying the pain nor its opposite. We are allowing both possibilities to be present, and we are therefore bringing ourselves back into balance. We often refer to this type of enquiry as an 'opposites practice' and it is quite a different approach to 'positive thinking' where we might focus only on the preferred outcome (i.e. 'It will definitely be OK') at the behest of recognising our very real fears and possibilities for the alternative.

So often when we feel unable to relax or struggle to unwind or even sleep, it's because we have entered into a frantic loop of worry: we become consumed by whatever it is that is troubling us, we try to push it away, or force it to take on a new shape, and it only comes back stronger and louder than before, and so it goes on. When we explore the opposite to that feeling or experience, rather than trying to convince ourselves that everything will be OK, or ignoring our fears, we are acknowledging our feelings while also bringing balance by recognising the possibility of the other extreme. We push nothing away, and we feel the very real possibility for things changing. As a result, without having 'resolved' the fear or having 'done anything' about it, typically, we are no longer dominated by it.

Enquiry 11:
Can you turn it around?

When we are somewhat overwhelmed by a particular thought, feeling, emotion or story about our life circumstance, it might be helpful to contemplate its opposite. Sometimes referred to as 'turning it around', it's important to recognise that this is not about getting *rid* of anything. When we reflect on an opposite sensation (relaxation vs tension), feeling (comfort vs pain), emotion (calm vs anxiety) or thought (I'm terrible at this vs I'm doing my best) it can help us to get 'unstuck'.

Whereas we might be much more drawn to feeling the opposite (who doesn't want to feel ease instead of pain!), this enquiry is about allowing *both* to be here. We are effectively neutralising the intensity of a particular experience; we are not denying its presence. We are allowing it, but we are recognising that we might need something to help us be present with it without being overwhelmed by it.

- Settle in to your most rested, nested position

- Allow some time to settle in. Be with what's arising. If you're feeling trapped in a story, notice how it makes you feel. What are the sensations you experience in your body as you welcome in this visitor? If we use the example of pain, what does it *actually* feel like?

- *Once you have a hold of how this feels (not thinking about the feeling, but the actual feeling), can you contemplate its opposite? For example, if you feel contraction in your belly, what might its opposite be? Stay with the felt sense of this, try not to figure out anything with your mind*

- *Once you've got a sense of the opposite sensation, can you move between the two? Rest your attention in one for a few moments, and then the other*

- *If you are able to do this, can you feel in to both of them at the same time? Your thinking mind cannot do this (it likes to divide and take sides) but by feeling them, you'll likely be able to feel both. Take your time. Don't rush it, or force anything*

- *If you have some insight or feelings of freedom or a new perspective, acknowledge the feeling of 'being'; that there is something here that's aware of these inner themes but that's not actually 'in' them. Remember the space between breaths from Enquiry 7 (see page 99) as a way to access that feeling of spaciousness and nothingness in which these sensations are occurring*

- *After a short while of feeling this quality of spaciousness, begin to transition from your time of rest. Wiggle your toes, have a little stretch, and notice the room around you*

- *Notice if you had any insights, feelings of freedom or new perspectives from this enquiry. See if you can loiter with that feeling as you move back in to your day*

Note: It may take you some time to get to an opposite. If we're really stuck on one thing, or aligned with a particular story, you might experience strong resistance to exploring its opposite. Remember that this is just one thing you can try, and it may be that any one of the other enquiries works just as well when facing a strong or overwhelming experience.

Even if your fears are realised, you can be OK

Sometimes, our worst fears *are* realised. This is a fact of life. How can we not be overwhelmed by such a possibility – especially when an unfortunate turn of events seems imminent? How can we still find a way to connect with that part of our being that is not thrown by catastrophe? How can the fact that we have no control over the situation and don't know how we will be affected by it bring a sense of relief?

If we consider the opposites practice in this situation (see *Enquiry 11: Can you turn it around?* on page 151), it doesn't rely on a change of circumstances to bring about a sense of balance. In order to not be overwhelmed by the fear, we bring in its opposite and allow it to be present in our experience at the same time. We are not denying our fear, merely bringing in a counter to it, so that we can 'be' with it without 'becoming' it.

In the same way, when it becomes inevitable that our worst fears really will play out, we can consider that while we will most likely experience extraordinary sadness and grief, we might also be able to cope with these feelings, and that we will, in time, feel OK again. We can ask such questions as:

'Is it true that I will not cope?'

Again, we cannot see into the future, so the answer can be, 'I do not *know* this to be true.'

We can then ask something such as, 'How might it feel to recover and move on from this event?' As we consider the answer, we can sense into a feeling of having gone through something difficult, while being able to continue to engage with and enjoy life once again. We can bring that feeling into the present alongside the worry, and we will most likely feel less overwhelmed by our fears, without refuting them.

'Everything will be OK' is not enough to help us find balance when extremely difficult events unfold in our lives – because everything is *not* OK. However, in the very worst of times, we can remind ourselves of the possibility that we are strong enough to cope. We may be changed, forever, but we might not be *broken* by the experience. As well as allowing your panic, shock or disappointment (whatever feelings are presenting themselves to you in the moment), if you can consider the possibility that you might be underestimating your ability to deal with those feelings, their power over you is countered without anything being denied.

While feeling thrown by events, you can also feel into the possibility that you are stronger than you imagined.

The very worst thing can happen, and, in time, you can be OK.

Just a whisper of this possibility might be all you need to catch a glimpse into your inherent, untouchable wholeness, and forever hold that glimpse within you as an experience – a remembering that at your most essential, you are OK.

ASK YOURSELF

Do you know how able to cope with something you are?
Can you entertain the possibility that you already have
everything you need within you to manage with even
the most upsetting turn of events?

Uncontrollable insight

As ever, we wish to draw your attention to a paradox to all this 'letting go' of seeking specific outcomes or of 'finding the positive': that when we accept that we cannot control outcomes, we might receive a most welcome outcome – something indeed very positive. On occasion, that feeling of ease, freedom and relaxation that comes from resting in not knowing brings about something new. A new way of seeing something or a spontaneous response can rise up out of we-don't-know-where. Having recognised what we think we know as nothing more than just that – a thought – we exist with a greater alertness to the present. We can see beyond our thoughts and our filters, and we are receptive to insight and epiphany.

We've all had moments when we've had a sudden realisation about a step to take, a wake-up call, a heartfelt feeling of super-confidence. Words fail to capture this innate knowing that has nothing to do with knowledge. It often comes without us having consciously worked anything out, or having sufficiently analysed a subject, or from accurately weighing up the pros and cons. None of these cerebral tasks were necessary to us having reached our truth. It just came, and it was clear.

ASK YOURSELF

Think of a time when you came to a sudden and deep knowing about something or someone? Can you describe exactly how that realisation presented itself to you?

Only we can know our truth, and it is only relevant to us. We can never ask someone else to help us find our truth, only perhaps help show us that we already know it.

Once we start trusting that we already know what is best for ourselves, and that this 'knowing' is not something we gain from research, interview or stretching our intellect, we can start to see what *is* over what we thought *might be*. We stop trying to control how we feel about something, and instead see how we really do feel about it.

We might find ourselves experiencing a new kind of wisdom, one that is less in the mind and more from our whole, deeper being.

This deeper knowing has a quieter quality; it's more of a whisper and less of a shout. We hear it only when we've turned all other noise down, and although it demands an acceptance of the unknowable qualities of life, it feels like the only truth.

When we stay connected to the infinite possibilities of life, and don't descend into that part of us that feels at odds with the world or that feels shame, guilt and personal responsibility when things go wrong – that part of us that is forever trying to find reason and excuses and opportunities to improve our behaviour – we can begin to see that our choices and actions can be informed from a deeper knowing that lies beyond the swirl of the mind. We are more able to feel into that part of our self that sees more clearly than our thoughts and knows more than our mind does. Even when a situation seems impossibly riddled with obstacles and complexities, we can resist the urge to set about the task of sorting it out and trust, instead, that part of us already knows the right response (for us).

Importantly, this isn't an exercise in 'self-knowledge' or stress management, or a practice in staying calm or any other taming of the mind. It's recognition that we can go beyond the mind and draw on an awareness that, even though unknown, exists as the only truth of any real value to us. Without rest – without ever stopping and relinquishing control – we are unable to experience ourselves beyond the stories of who we are, what we want and what we can do. We must go beyond the stories, and beyond control, to see ourselves completely.

Engaging, not escaping

Amid the communities in which we work and play – largely yoga and meditation – we frequently come across individuals who embrace the practices of these traditions as a means to escape from their experience of life rather than to engage with it. We might even have felt this way ourselves in the past: you find a lifestyle that removes all so-called 'bad' things from your life, be that 'bad' foods, 'bad' habits, 'bad' thoughts or those famous 'toxic friends', and you soon feel rested and at ease. Suddenly life seems manageable again. But we would argue that you might have actually removed *life* from your experience.

We've both spent considerable lengths of time in ashrams, which to the uninitiated are typically institutions where you live under dictated conditions – from the time you get up, to what you can eat, to how you practise yoga and meditation. The experience leaves you feeling incredible: your body feels amazing, your mind clear and your nervous system calm. You've had all obstacles removed. You've had the everyday stresses of making any decisions for yourself removed, and you've not had the stimulation of technology or angst of social networking or indeed any networking. You've been gentle on yourself and the environment has been gentle to you. It's an amazing experience, and afterwards we've both had a momentary thought that we have somehow found the best way to live.

All we have to do is remove pretty much everything from our old lives. . .

The most we've managed is perhaps being vegetarian for a couple of months, but both of us have found that our bodies breathe a massive sigh of relief when we take a first bite out of that much-denied beef burger.

For most of us, these 'pure' lifestyles are simply not sustainable. Not unless you commit to leaving your old life behind and forever living like a monk (or indeed, do become a monk). For some people, this is the choice that they make, and they go on to live under restrained conditions in an institution where they do not engage with the outside world. Everything is controlled for them. If this is your calling, then good for you. But most of us do want to continue to live in the society from which we came and spend time with our friends and family, and so we have to find a way to live amid obstacles, challenges and temptations. We have to learn to be with the trappings of everyday life without feeling that we constantly have to resist them. We have to be bold enough to admit when we're feeling bad, both to ourselves and to others, otherwise we will be left exhausted by the alternative: denial, running away, hiding, forcing, resisting. We also want to be able to live a life that involves risks and challenges – we don't want to hide from life as a means to protect ourselves from ever feeling pain. We have to expect and allow mistakes, misfortune, disappointment and stress in our experience; this is the deal with engaging in the world and everyone in it.

Rest is the ultimate act of allowing everything to be just as it is. It is not dependent on anything other than a surrendering of control, desire and condition. Rest has no conditions. If you find yourself trying to control rest, remind yourself that if there is one thing you need to do about your restlessness, it's nothing.

Rest and Your Self

We might now be starting to see how our preoccupation with controlling our lives and controlling our feelings about our lives is taking us away from just *being* in our lives. As we stop and experience who we are when we are not controlling, acquiring or working anything out, we see a self that is beyond definition. When we rest – when we are inhabiting only our awareness – we have no name, no desires, no status and the physical makeup of our body is irrelevant. In this way, in those moments of pure awareness, there is nothing to differentiate us from anyone else. Our self is in many ways, insignificant.

You might find this an uncomfortable proposition, and it stands against so much of what we are presented as being the key to a 'good' and 'well' life – self-care, self-improvement, self-help. It's easy to see why so many of us see it our duty to take our 'self', understand it, tame it, define and refine it.

But being able to step back from the concept of your 'self' and step into something greater – something indefinable, unimprovable and always *well* (something that *is* literally your wellbeing) – is the very nature of rest. It is a relinquishing of all self-concern and a surrendering into what remains beyond. When we rest, we experience ourselves beyond any ideas, hopes or criticisms we have about ourselves. We see that we are still there, regardless.

Therefore, our desire to know ourselves, from the experiences of our childhood to the habits we find ourselves caught up in today, might be in the way of us truly knowing ourselves. This might be what is preventing us from stepping back into who we are beyond all definition and explanation.

Stepping back from your experiences and your responses to them

How we behave and respond to the events that shape our lives is down to countless factors, some inherent and some not. We have our genetic makeup, our inherent human programming, and then there are the external factors, such as how we were raised, how we were treated and the events of our lives to date. We are all incredibly complex and we could spend years trying to unpick our roots and understand why we do the things we do and feel the things we feel, but we'll never reach a conclusion or be certain of any particular explanation. You might have had parents who never praised you, but that might not the reason you seek reassurance from your partner. You might come from a family of strong, fearless business people, but that might not be why you're so good at managing projects and negotiating deals. The reason you are so brave in terrifying circumstances could be down to a particular mindset you've worked hard to achieve, but it could also be for reasons completely out of your control, such as your genes.

You cannot know yourself in terms of cause and effect, and very often why you do the things you do has nothing to do with 'you'. You did not make you happen. If we consider our inherent behaviour traits then we know that the way we respond and react to life is somewhat hardwired into us. We all have some basic programming that drives how we live, and this is not our fault or necessarily something we should seek to understand. It's simply the way we are.

For example, when we feel attacked in some way, either physically or psychologically (a car we are travelling in skids out of control, we have a gun pulled on us, someone hurls shocking abuse at us), most of us, in the first instance, will freeze. This reaction comes not from our upbringing or previous experiences or from choice, but out of a very basic mechanism deep in the stem of our brain that learned to play dead when in danger. You might not like this or other aspects of how you respond to various situations, but there might be very little you can do about it, and perhaps more importantly, not much to be gained from trying to analyse such behaviours.

Analysis and therapy can certainly help us to explore and navigate ourselves, or even just help us take a look at ourselves, but you can also consider and take relief from the possibility that you exist beyond the stories of your life and the detail of your makeup.

When you rest, you might see that at the deepest level, you transcend the details of your life and your programming.

Your essential self – that 'awareness' we dissolve into when we are resting – bears no relation to any of the stories, explanations or beliefs you hold for how you think and behave.

— When you are resting, or otherwise catching a glimpse of your essential self, you are not engaging in thought about who you are, you simply are.

There is nothing about who you are that you can control or understand any better in that moment. There is no judgement or assessment. There is no story. . . and yet, there you are.

You will see that you exist beyond the history and narrative of your life, and you might be able to take solace in the possibility that there is no mystery to be solved here. You might prefer that things were different, but you might be less attached to the idea of having to make it so. Any feelings of shame or inadequacy about who you are might start to lessen. You might also start feeling the same way about other people.

To try to understand why we act the way we do and feel the way we do is like entering a maze that has no exit. It might be an interesting adventure, with some unexpected twists and turns, but there is no conclusion or, ultimately, any way out. While this kind of self-knowledge and understanding has some value, you can never truly hold a picture that accurately depicts why you are the way you are. As much as this may be frustrating, it also means you are free from any obligation you may have felt to figure yourself out. Instead, you can pay witness to how you are feeling within experiences as they happen, and instead of asking 'why?' you are feeling the way you do, you can listen to your feelings and respond with the kind of clarity that can only come when all filters are off.

The story of you is not who you are, and therefore you do not need to know the ins and the outs of every narrative. Ultimately, self-knowledge cannot be acquired or learned, it can only be experienced. For many of us, this is a radical proposition, and perhaps even as awkward as it is appealing – you are never going to find the answer to the question of you. Your thoughts about you, your feelings about you, and your inherent programming are not components that add up to make you, and some of them shift and change and develop and disappear. Yet 'you' carry on regardless.

If you are inclined to seek out explanations for why you are 'you', it might be interesting to ask yourself what your motive is for doing this. What's driving you? Do you feel there is something missing from 'you'? What do you think will happen when you find the missing piece of the apparent puzzle? Do you think 'not knowing' yourself is unusual? Can you lean into the possibility that none of us 'knows' ourselves via knowledge? Who is the 'you' who wants to know about yourself?

Working with a therapist, for example, can offer wonderful insight and presents an invaluable forum for us to share our feelings and experiences in a way that we might not want, or feel able, to with friends and family. As we explore our inner world, memories and perhaps even dreams, we might develop a sense of self-trust, but rarely will it provide conclusions – the 'story' of your own self-narrative can never be 'done', for you exist beyond the story.

ASK YOURSELF

What do you find most puzzling about yourself?
How do feel about the possibility of never understanding this aspect of yourself? Does it change who you are?

Enquiry 12:
Can you let go of the stories about yourself?

We all have a sense of separate self. We all have a narrative in our heads and, accompanying it, a feeling of being separate. It's part of what makes us human. The good news? It's just another set of thoughts and feelings that you can become aware of.

In this enquiry we invite you to go on the search for yourself. Can you find one, consistent voice among your inner dialogue? Can you locate, as a feeling or sensation, the place where 'you' are? Or, instead, is there something in your experience that stays the same, while all else shifts and changes? Is there something *behind* the search for you? And if so, what, where, how and who is it?

- *Settle in, get ready to let it all go*

- *For a few moments do nothing but embrace everything just as it is. No pushing away. No clinging on. No need to work anything out. No need to get anywhere*

- *Now, ask yourself, 'Where am I?' Can you find a location for your sense of self?*

- *As you watch different thoughts, perceptions and images come and go, ask yourself where do they come from? Is there a 'somebody', a sense of self producing these experiences? Or are they just happening?*

- As self-talk appears, can you notice if there's a central orchestrator to this narrative? Does it seem like one voice, or many different ones? Are they all in harmony? Is there a consistency?

- While you watch all this come and go and move and change, can you find a quality that is unchanging and familiar?

- As you find this unchanging quality, is there a voice here? A narrative? Or is it more of a quiet watchfulness? Is this place that seems consistent full of beliefs, stories and ideas, or is it the place in which all these stories appear?

- Stay for as long as feels fruitful. Notice how you feel. Is it scary, or liberating? How do you feel about finding (or losing) your sense of self? Is your thinking mind confused?

- When you feel ready to, begin to transition from this quiet time into activity. Wiggle your fingers and toes, stretch, move in a way that's spontaneous and natural. Take your time, especially if you feel a bit spaced out

Rest and separation

Most of the time we go about our lives with a very fixed sense of isolation – it's 'us' against the world. This is a natural part of our self-recognition mechanism – essentially our in-built navigation system. It gives the perception of there being an 'us' in here (our body) and a 'them' or 'it' out there – other people, the world and everything we perceive and take in through our senses. This sense of division contributes to our sense of 'struggle' and suffering: we feel separate from our environment and therefore seek to control it, manipulate it and get hold of more of what we like about it and get rid of that which we don't like.

But what if this sense of separation is nothing more than a device – an illusion? What if you were not separate from any of it? What if you really were always 'at one with the universe'?

Our sense of being 'in here' can quite quickly dissipate by asking the question, where is this 'me' located? You might have a feeling of being 'inside your head', but is there one overruling sense of who you are 'in there'?

We can talk about our body, we can talk about our thoughts, dreams and hopes, but when we ask *where* are we, we cannot pin it down to any one place or any one central figure. There seems to be a clamour of different voices and opinions and ideas but no chief orchestrator. (If there were one, wouldn't we be able to pull all of our disparate ideas and thoughts together into a cohesive whole?)

Science is yet to define one area – one place in the brain area – where our self-narrative comes from. So far, the closest thing to be identified is a network of areas that light up in the brain when we talk about ourselves. Different parts of the brain come together to help us process, decide, discriminate and judge, but there is no known central 'I' to it. It's a collection of systems that perceive a fixed point in time and a fixed location, but there's no ultimate 'I'.

So, if you're not in your brain, and if you're not in your body, then where are you?

ASK YOURSELF

You probably have a sense that there's a somebody, most likely up there in your head, taking everything in. What if you took a moment to explore this 'somebody'. Can you feel where they are? Do they feel like a thing, or a space? Is it hard, or soft? Limited, or unlimited? Where does it begin and end?

As you explore 'where' you are, you might notice fewer limits to this 'you'. And even though there may still be part of your brain function insisting that it is the 'you' located somewhere within your body, you might now be able to feel into the possibility that this particular voice is not 'you' – and that you are not as limited as this concept of 'you'. You have a thinking brain, which tries to figure everything out and provide a framework for your existence, but you expand beyond this concept. You are more than this.

Enquiry 13:
What is happening in your body?

Even when you are still, your body is moving. Whether you believe in such a thing as 'life force' (or 'vital force', 'qi' or 'ch'i') as long as you are alive, your body is energised, and so we have the opportunity to witness the effects of energy in the body.

Setting about this observation is one of the most powerful practices we use as a means to help people see themselves and their body in a way they never have before.

In previous enquiries you might have observed your body and your breath, and noticed how they regulate themselves, and how turning your attention to sensation instead of thought can induce an unconscious release of tension. These are all ways that might help you to see that you don't need to 'figure out' how to rest, but that it happens *to* you. Now you can go even further and deeper with this idea by watching how your body is being breathed (and doing everything it needs to do) but consider that this is not necessarily by 'you'.

As you observe your breath you will feel your belly swelling and moving and your chest expanding and contracting. If you pay attention for long enough, you might notice your shoulders being subtly moved by your rib cage, and your pelvis and hips being moved by the movement in the belly. As you pay closer attention you might feel how the arms and legs are also responding to the breath.

You might then begin to notice your whole body breathing, or at least feel how every last element of it responds to the breath. No part of you remains still.

We can take this a stage further still: as you follow those subtle sensations of movement, you might begin to feel how the whole body is alive with sensation, from your fingers to your toes. Your body feels vibrant; not a static and solid object but a subtle flow of endless sensation.

At this point, we might feel how the breath, the body and all our sensations not only seem less defined but also less personal – less *ours*. They are movement without limits, outside of our control, somehow holding us and somehow independent of us, too.

This can be at once mesmerising and surprising, as we feel the body at this level it's hard to believe it's the same thing you see when you look in the mirror.

- *Make yourself comfortable, sitting or lying, and close your eyes*

- *Observe the breath. Notice as it comes in and goes out. Do not alter this movement (do not stop it from altering either. . .)*

- *Notice where you feel your breath. Is it in your belly? Throat? Nostrils?*

- *Keep observing and watching where you feel the effects of your breath*

- Open out your attention to include more and more of the body. How are these parts of your body responding?

- Keep moving and observing around the body

- Ask yourself if there is any part of your body *not* responding to the breath?

- Notice, throughout your body, if any sensations feel fixed

- Are you mostly static, or mostly dynamic (even if on a micro-level)?

- Stay observing your body, its movements, the switching out of these movements, the greater movements, the tiniest exchanges. Feel every happening of your body

- Rest with the sensations of your body for as long as you wish

- When you're ready, transition back from noticing sensation to creating it by gently moving your body and bring yourself back to wakefulness

Switching off from 'you'

When you stop and rest, your mind starts to slow down, and with little new information coming in to your brain through your senses you become more aware of other aspects of your experience, such as bodily sensations and feelings. It might take a while for your brain to calm down, as there could be leftovers of memory and other things from your day moving through (this is the chatter that we've reassured you is perfectly OK and not a hindrance to rest), but by and by, there will be a slowing down, a quietening that will naturally unfold. As this happens to you (without effort), and especially if you've been entering rest more 'consciously' (the effect is cumulative), you might start to sense the possibility that you are not a consciousness inhabiting a body, but something subtler with no discernible boundary. You become aware of the possibility that where you begin and other things end is blurred.

The mechanisms of our mind that positions us as a separate entity relax when we're not engaging with the world; that is, when we stop – when we are resting. Manoeuvring around objects, talking to someone or scrolling through social media newsfeeds will bring us into a deeper sense of 'me' over here and 'it' (or them) over there. In contrast, when we do nothing (absolutely nothing), this natural brain function relaxes. We don't need to navigate the world when we rest, and so our navigation tools switch off. We no longer see ourselves as having to make our way through the world because the world is us.

This is a massive concept to take in – but you don't have to. You can merely contemplate it as a *possibility* and then you might fall, without effort, into a greater sense of self – into a feeling of the magnificence of being total. That rather than living in the world, you *are* the world. Whenever you're facing a challenge or feeling bad about who you are and what you're going through, you can step back (or perhaps even step in) and consider how, ultimately, you might be a contributing part of something immense and incredible.

You can also consider when you might already have previously sensed into this possibility by chance. Perhaps you can recall a moment from your childhood when you had a feeling of being part of everything – or subtler, that you did not see yourself as separate.

Another starting point might be to simply contemplate the air you breathe. Breathing comprises a constant exchange between our surroundings and ourselves. Through our breath we are connected, inexorably, with the world around us. The air that you are now breathing was, at one point, on the other side of the earth. The carbon dioxide that you exhale as part of your next breath out has the potential to become a flower in another part of the world. Part of what you are right now, was once another living organism – a tree, flower or planet – giving its life to sustain yours. As you breathe, you are part of *everything*.

Our sense of self is very firmly rooted in what we see in the mirror: an object within the world. We see ourselves as being 'in' our body and our environment and other people 'out there'. As we go about our day-to-day lives, we do so with this picture of ourselves as a disparate being. A great deal of our suffering can come from this feeling of being separate. It's us against the world. We're alone. We're not part of anything – or we're not good enough to contribute. When we feel our separateness more strongly, we're less able to relate to other people.

When we express ourselves as feeling 'safe in our own skin', we typically mean that we accept and feel good about who we are and the situation we find ourselves in. But our skin, interestingly, is what we think of as holding us 'in' and separating us from the world.

In this enquiry, we take a moment to draw our attention to this perceived boundary and observe what really happens at the point at which we think we end and everything else begins. Do we sense a firm line between the world and us? If not, what do we notice?

When we rest, our sense of separation dissolves. We aren't even aware of our body. When we rest our unconditioned attention on the place where we perceive our separation to be, this separation might become less distinct. We might not even sense there to be one at all. We have an opportunity to feel ourselves as not being bound by our skin but as something that has no border, something spacious and inherently interconnected with everything in our experience and beyond.

This enquiry is best explored if you have experimented with swapping thought for sensation (*Enquiry 3: What happens if you turn your attention from thought to sensation?* on page 46) and observed the endless dance of aliveness and fluid sensations that make up the body (*Enquiry 13: What is happening in your body?* on page 46).

- *Find yourself some time and space in which to do nothing. You can practise with lying down or sitting up, and it's best to close your eyes*

- *Once comfortable, turn your attention to the mass of sensations that make up your body. Notice how your body is alive, shifting and changing*

- *Don't take our word for it though. Be with your body until you can feel its vibrant aliveness. You can start by observing the breath and how it makes your body move, then extend out, watching the endless movements and responses*

- *Now, rest your attention on the feeling of the front of your body. Notice it in relationship to any surfaces, clothing and air that it touches*

- *Remind yourself that your intention must be to feel not think your way to finding the place where your body ends and the surfaces, clothing and air begin*

- Take your time with this. Don't rush to find a conclusion. Stay open to your experience

- Now do the same with feeling the back of your body

- Then feel the left side, in relationship to what lies beyond, and then the right side

- Now feel all directions at the same time: above, below, left, right. Keep *feeling* your way into the place where you end and your surroundings begin

- Spend a few moments just being with whatever you sense. Rest in it for as long as possible, without thinking about it

- When you're ready, bring your attention back to your breath, move your body gently, and come back to wakefulness (or wherever you were before you started this enquiry)

Rest and death

However you see your self, your experience of being in the body you are in right now, with your memories and sensations and preferences and passions, will end. Of this, we can be sure. Whatever your beliefs about your soul, your being, your spirit, you know that your body will someday die.

Many cultures meditate (or 'focus' to be more accurate) on death in explicit detail, from visualising their festering body to imagining their skeleton and even that skeleton dissolving into dust. This might seem like a sure-fire way to bring about misery, but it is perhaps one of the most potent 'acceptance' practices there is. If you can *be* with the knowledge of your demise, then you are at peace with perhaps the most difficult aspect of life – that it ends – and you are at the same time making yourself aware of the value of your living presence right now.

Do most of us live day-to-day in denial that we are going to die, or in acceptance? Perhaps we oscillate between the two, but either way it is a fact that, for most of us most of the time, death is rarely at the forefront of our awareness. Our impending death is not something we like to think about, and so when such a thought does enter our experience, as it can do at the most peculiar of times, most of us tend to push it away for fear that it will make us unhappy. Perhaps we are missing an opportunity here to meet a valuable messenger, one who can bring us back to ourselves when we feel distracted, frantic or bemoaning of our situation and desiring *more*.

As we remember the inevitability of our own death, we might change our priorities, or we might gain a new perspective on an old issue. We might honour the preciousness of every moment just a little bit more, whether we're feeling low or happy, at least we are *feeling something*.

Rest and Your Future

Have you ever said to yourself, 'I should be more present'? It is a widely held belief that thinking too much about what has happened in the past or worrying about what might happen in the future brings suffering in the present moment. For this reason, it's become popular to use practices and techniques intended to pull our attention back to the here and now. You might have tried to consciously notice what is happening around you, from the subtlest of sounds, physical sensations and minute details of your environment. You might have focused on your breath. You might have taken pen to paper and coloured in an intricate drawing.

With any of these kinds of mindfulness practices, you might notice your thoughts become quieter, your emotions less overwhelming and your worries about tomorrow ease off. You find a sense of feeling centred and of being less at the mercy of your sometimes-turbulent mind and the frenzy of your everyday life. They are excellent practices. However, perhaps we might be missing something important here: perhaps, by declaring ourselves 'not present' and then applying a practice to make us present, we are missing the presence that is *always* present.

Again, we are setting about a task with the intention of getting somewhere; by trying to *make* ourselves 'live in the moment' we are pronouncing ourselves to be somewhere not as good as where we could be. We run the risk of forgetting that, essentially, we are always exactly where we should be.

ASK YOURSELF

If you have a formal meditation or mindfulness practice, can you approach the technique from the perspective that you are always present? As you begin, make note of your intention and remind yourself that don't need to go looking for presence, or make yourself 'do it'. It is already happening.

When are you?

Whatever you are thinking right now, is happening right now.

That memory you're having, you're having it right now.

That fear about the future? That's your present fear.

You are not a time traveller. You are always present.

But, of course, that's not to say you don't have thoughts that distract you from this fact. When we rest and when we catch glimpses of our innate unwavering being, we are not self-reflecting or running a commentary, analysing or interpreting. We have no concept of past, present or future. As we experience our awareness, we are not any more or any less present than at any other time. We are directly experiencing our existence beyond any such concepts.

Your essential self is impervious to any thoughts you have about time, and any constructs that as a society we use to order the past, present and future. It is timeless.

ASK YOURSELF

Can you reflect on a feeling of 'being'? That quality of being absorbed in something beautiful or captivating, or experiencing a fleeting moment of crystal-clear awareness (this can come in times of stress, it is not dependent on 'positive' environmental factors)? As you were in this 'glimpse' of pure being, what time was it? Were you even aware of time?

When we approach any of the techniques we think of as practices to help us be 'more present' we can instead remind ourselves that they are not making us any *more* present, but helping us to see that we are always present.

And if you ever find yourself declaring 'I must be more present' in your everyday life, perhaps a more useful declaration would be (even when reaching for your smartphone) 'I am always present'. And as you say those words, you remind yourself of, and rest back into, your inherent constant awareness (and you'll probably be less interested in that Instagram feed from that person who likes to tell you how to be more present. . .).

— *We are not in the past, we are not in the future, we are present.*

Giving up your future self

When we are not feeling rested, we might hope that our most rested, contented self will manifest in the future once we've got all our rest 'done'.

We are both right and wrong in this imagining: when we rest in being (which we can do right now), we don't think about the future, because we are resting in that place (that 'everywhere') where everything is always still, quiet and in need of nothing. But the echoes of this experience will mean that even when we are not resting, our mind will be more relaxed (not because we've made it so, it's just an outcome of doing nothing) and we will find ourselves less fixated on the need to know what the future holds to the level of fine detail.

As we become more familiar with our awareness, we come to realise that it is not necessary – or possible – for us to know how to create the future that we think we want. We realise that what we think might make us feel happier (or safer, or more at ease) in the future is only ever a thought.

What's more, as we become further aware of these glimpses of our 'completeness', we come to know that they are unconditional. In short, we see how unreliable the future is, and we are able to loosen our grip on it as a place where we have everything arranged just as we think we wish it to be. We see how what is happening right now is held by something utterly contented, something that isn't missing or lacking in anything.

We use the framework of time to organise our thoughts, and importantly, prepare for the future. You put a date in your diary, the event comes around, you experience that event, and then you have a memory of that event. However, although we know that what we do now will have implications for our experiences to come, we have little idea what our future experiences will be like and particularly how we will feel about them at the time.

This gives us the opportunity to loosen our investment in the future as a place where we will have found the things we feel are missing from our present. If we can recognise that our vision of how our future might look and how we will feel as a result is nothing more than a fantastic projection, then we might find it easier to stop investing in it as a place where we will be a better version of who we are right now. We cannot 'be' more in the future than we 'are' right now.

Throughout the book we've taken time to outline a recurrent message: that what you are looking for is already here. Your rested self is already the case.

This understanding is not something that can come in time. The understanding is always here. Sometimes (by stopping) you glimpse it; sometimes you feel it because all else just so happens to be absent. It is definitely not waiting for you at some point in the future.

You are looking for the glasses that are on top of your head.

ASK YOURSELF

How important to you is the idea that your future will be easier than your present?

This will always be the conundrum: you cannot realise a more ease-filled existence if you believe it exists in the future. That rested self, that quiet-essence that's beyond the mind, is not dependent on you doing anything at all. It's right here. Right now. If it is not here now, then it cannot be in the future.

Even we, the 'rest experts' (we can be bold enough to proclaim ourselves expert at nothing!) often have to remind ourselves that what we are desiring is already here, and what a joyful reminder this can be! The challenge is that with this reminder – as we rest, stop, allow for a glimpse of the inner stillness that is our home ground of being – we have to be prepared to do something brave. We have to completely *give up* the future. We must set fire to it. We must see it as separate to our ability to feel rested, to feel at-peace, to feel at one with our lives.

In order to bring ourselves into the possibility that our rested self is not something we can work towards for the future (if we do enough 'being' and the right kind of 'letting go'), we can see how it might feel to let go of the insistence that what we are looking for is *not* here already.

ASK YOURSELF

How do you feel about the future when you contemplate that a more restful experience of life is not dependent on either external circumstances or internal developments?

When we rest, we are unaware of time and we are unaware of any boundaries, we are infinite and timeless. The future plays no part in us realising this.

Rest and ambition

It is perfectly reasonable to have dreams for the future, and it is perfectly reasonable to have fears for the future, but we should perhaps accept that they are no more than thoughts and, whether they come true or not, we don't know how we're going to feel as a result of them manifesting or not. As much as this leaves us at the mercy of fate (or whatever you wish to call the unfolding of events and experiences), it also demonstrates how we are not bound into anything being one way or another. We are free.

We are all growing, learning and developing. We are not static in any way. It's impossible not to learn and grow as our life unfolds and we gather experience, knowledge and understanding. This growth potential is essential to our lives and it is not in conflict with what we are sharing in this book. Next year, you will be facing new circumstances and reacting in a different way to them than you would today.

Our actions cause an effect and throughout the course of our lives we will have choices to make and opportunities to grasp. Therefore, we have a responsibility to ourselves and to the world in which we live to consider how our actions might affect the future. However, our experience of the future – how it will look, how we will feel, how others will respond to it – is not something we have very much control over at all. We are in this way constantly dancing between intending to do that which will have the best outcome for everyone, while accepting that we will inevitably be surprised. We cannot 'win' and we cannot 'lose' – we are not bound into the outcome. We are, in effect, all passengers on a train being driven by everyone all at once. Although the destination is unknowable, we can both take pleasure in the drive itself as well as our vision of reaching a pleasant destination.

None of us knows the best way to live, but we are all entitled to explore what motivates us, what excites and inspires us, and share this with the world without it being conditional on the world responding in a particular way, or the future (destination) taking a particular shape because of it. As we take a moment to rest, to stop everything and let go of any intention, desire or expectations, we experience that part of us that is timeless, spacious and without preference, and our need for the future to be a particular way is slackened.

This might not change what we do or what we campaign for, but it might bring ease into a place where otherwise there was only a sense of being on the 'offensive', which is far from anything we have been discussing in this book: balance, awareness, spaciousness, harmony, stillness and presence.

Does the idea that you are not as in control of your future as you might think bring you a sense of relief or make you feel anxious? How does this notion relate to your current beliefs about your future?

As humans, we have opinions and preferences and we will want to shape our future according to our ideals. However, it is possible to act, share and assert them without it being some form of an attack, either on an institution, an ideology or ourselves. Indeed, throughout this book we have been bringing aspects of cultural, spiritual, societal and even religious belief into question, though at no point have we attacked these beliefs. We know that we don't know it all – that nobody does.

— We must be humbled by the unarguable mysteriousness of life.

When planning for our future, we must be open to the possibility that the outcome of our planning might surprise us. Things on the surface might seem better than they do now, or worse, and either way, we remain as complete as we always were. We are in this way, future-proof.

You probably have a natural inclination to see the future as a place where you are a better version of yourself. We all do this, all the time, and that's largely OK and has its benefits (drive, ambition, creativity, causes), but in this enquiry we might see how our preoccupation with our future self might be doing a disservice to our current self and the life it is living right now. If we imagine that we will be 'better' in the future, we might not be 'bothering' so much about today – we put ourselves on hold.

However, this is not our call for you to be 'more present'. Your thoughts, feelings and memories always appear in the present moment. In this way, you can't be any more 'present' than you already are. However, you may not be aware of this fact, and you might be missing an opportunity to enjoy this fact. Through rest we do not necessarily make ourselves any more 'mindful' or any more 'present' but we do have an opportunity to see that we have a wholeness to us – an essence of completeness – that is as perfect and at peace now as it will be in the future. This is the only thing we can be sure of.

In this enquiry we focus on letting go of our idealised future, not by getting away from it or seeing it as a distraction, but by realising it as a non-sense, something that we cannot ever be sure about, something we can never really know. We're seeing through it completely and setting fire to it as a notion (for a short while). We are honouring the fact that there is no grander version of awareness waiting for us in the future. The belief that we might one day be more able to fully embrace our deeper nature could be the very thing keeping us locked away from it.

- *Set yourself up for rest in a way that works for you (or try something new. . .)*

- *As you settle, take on the stance that there is no 'future you'. We invite you for just moments to let go of the idea that you will be more anything in the future (more rested, more peaceful, more content, more fulfilled)*

- *Instead, enquire into whether or not you might sense a quality to your experience right now that already feels rested, peaceful, content and fulfilled. As you rest right now, might you feel into a sense of ease that is already here, right behind you, in front of you and all around?*

- *Consider how it could be that the only part of your experience that will ever feel fully this way is already here. It's not a future project, but something to rest into right now, something to bask in and feel deeply fulfilled by. It is something that already knows perfection and timelessness and it has plenty of space. It needs nothing to feel whole and complete*

- *As you rest in this way, you might become distracted by counter thoughts and sensations – don't try to get away from* any of it. Feel that everything is included in this wholeness. There's nowhere to get to, no way that this aspect of your experience needs to be more 'mindful'. It's already perfectly present and completely rested

- Stay with this sense of timeless completeness for a few moments – preferably, for minutes

- Thoughts will come and go and that's OK, just keep returning to the space in which they are held

- When you are ready, take a breath, stretch/wriggle and resurface

Why you cannot create a more rested version of yourself in the future

Rest requires nothing; it does not need you to invest in anything now to ensure you are able to do it tomorrow. Rest is always here; it might be the only thing that remains within the possibility of your experience at all times.

You cannot earn, buy, develop or nourish rest. It makes no sense to sacrifice rest so that you might rest in the future.

If you do not have time to take more rest than you do already, then observe the natural pauses in your day – however momentary. Watch them. Allow them to be there. All your busy-ness plays out within a spaciousness that never leaves you. This space is limitless, and it's here right now.

. . . and Sleep

In writing a book about rest, we cannot ignore the subject of sleep. It's become a topic of enormous interest and discourse, with countless books, blog pieces, magazine articles and television documentaries on the subject. The jury is out as to whether this is because we're getting less sleep than ever before, are feeling a greater sense of tiredness/fatigue/stress, or simply have more information and the technology to better understand the science of sleep.

We can't tell you that rest can replace sleep. It can't. But when you're low on sleep you can help yourself enormously by paying attention to how you rest (or don't rest). You've probably heard the expression, 'sleep begets sleep', but we would like to add that *rest* also begets sleep, and it goes the other way, too.

When we sleep well at night we experience a glorious list of advantages: happier disposition, improved digestion (and we're better able to discern the right type and amount of food that we really need), we feel at ease in our body, with reduced muscle tension, more patience, and a general feeling of being able to cope better with whatever life throws our way. We enter into an upward spiral, where the fact that we feel rested and whole allows us to continue to feel rested and whole.

However, for many of us a good night's sleep is the exception and not the rule, and so by turning our attention to rest we can experience a two-fold benefit. First, we find some immediate relief in the process of being witness to that part of us that is always OK (regardless of the sleep deprivation); secondly, the sleep that we do get will most likely be sounder and come more easily.

Are you obsessed with sleep?

We know that sleep plays an exceptional role in our ability to function as balanced, healthy, rational, emotionally intelligent individuals. It is the ultimate healer, soother, refresher, reviver and reformer. It's even one of our most inventive creative aides, with dreams offering inspiration and a well-rested brain the ability to string more than two sentences together. A bad night's sleep can ruin a day; a good night's sleep can make it. When hosting a guest overnight, the first thing we want to know is whether or not they slept well (to which the correct response is always, 'Yes', at which point said guest must be supplied with at least two large cups of coffee, regardless).

Sleep is something that some of us claim to do 'like a baby' (although if you have ever had a baby you will be baffled by this comparison), while others declare themselves bad sleepers, waking frequently and not being able to take themselves back off (like an actual baby, perhaps). Some of us recognise that we are night owls, at our happiest staying up into the small hours, while others boast about being up with the lark, though unable to stay up much past 10 p.m. Some of us believe we don't sleep well at all, while our partners claim to have heard us snoring since the early hours.

Perhaps you lust after the weekend so you can indulge in that extra-long lie-in, or maybe you struggle with sleep so much you can't stand your bedroom or anything that reminds you of those hours spent awake tossing and turning and willing the morning to come.

— For some of us, what should be the most restful activity in our life brings us the most stress.

Whatever your current relationship with sleep, you've probably now heard of the term 'sleep hygiene' – perhaps it's even now on your bedtime to-do list. Every day new sleep-tracking gadgets and apps appear on the market, and more and more claims regarding sleep's importance are asserted, and experts appear and case studies are presented and counter-studies and research papers and. . .

It's exhausting.

So, what are we to do with all this information?

Sleep might be completely out of your control

We once listened to a frazzled mother who, when bemoaning how little sleep she was getting, confessed she had begun to fantasise about having a minor road accident just serious enough to warrant a stay in hospital and, what she longed for, uninterrupted time to sleep. Of course, she was not *entirely* serious, but it does demonstrate just how desperate extreme tiredness can leave us feeling.

For many of us, how and why we sleep the way we do remains mysterious and unpredictable. Sometimes we fluke a great night of zeds, other times we put everything in place to ensure The Sandman performs his duties, and for some reason he never shows up. And for some of us a good night's sleep is straight-up unattainable regardless of how good our sleep hygiene is. Illness, pregnancy, small children, big children, noisy neighbours – these are all things completely out of our control that can disturb our sleep.

Typically, worrying about anything isn't conducive to a good night's sleep. Therefore, surrounding yourself in literature that relays just how very vital it is for your health that you do sleep, while you continue to battle either a mystifying sleep condition or something out of your control that keeps waking you up, is not likely to help.

You have a problem that you already know is a problem and then you are simply equipping yourself with more information that confirms how bad your problem is. This is a problem.

If you are tired, everything can seem like a problem. So, when it comes to sleep, perhaps you should start by considering the possibility that rather than a problem that requires fixing you might simply have a situation that needs nothing more than your attention, at least in the first instance. The former requires us knowing how to resolve a situation, whereas the latter requires no more than the awareness we already have (or, the awareness we already are).

Becoming aware of how you feel about sleep

Seeing as you have chosen to read a book about rest, we can assume you are experiencing, to a certain extent, tiredness in your life right now. How do you feel about that?

As a society, we're very keen to express how busy we are, but not so quick to bemoan our tiredness apart from to those whom we feel especially close. Very few people would inform their boss, for example, that they are completely exhausted. We want to be seen as bright and capable, and in this way tiredness has become a matter of shame (one obvious exception to this is new parents, who are 'allowed' to feel tired at all times – it actually becomes 'news' when you are not tired). Very often, we keep our fatigue under wraps, or cover it up with that extra cup of coffee or the latest beauty products designed to make us look radiant.

This covering up is one of the first places we might look to get an insight into our relationship with sleep, seeking to identify just how much we mask our tiredness. Are we doing this for ourselves as much as anyone else? Perhaps we weren't even aware that we were doing this particularly, it's just become part of our routine.

If we realise that we are ignoring or masking over our tiredness, it might be interesting to stop and listen to what our body might be telling us. What might we learn if we stop masking our fatigue and instead engage with it? This could be an obvious and clear way to start a self-enquiry, to recognise what it means to stop and observe what's really going on with you right now. The important thing is to pay attention to how you are feeling rather than immediately try to figure out how to fix it. Obsessing over sleep does not induce sleep, whereas observing how you think and feel about sleep might. And if it doesn't, at least you will feel less tension alongside your tiredness.

ASK YOURSELF

Are you tired right now? If so, where do you feel it? Is it physical, mental? Both? How have you been dealing with it? Why?

The difference between fixing and tending to

If you've ever found yourself in the depths of sleep deprivation then you'll know how all-consuming a state it is. All you can think about is the fact you are tired and all you can talk about is the fact you are tired. Every aspect of your experience is filtered through the lens of sleeplessness. The gloss is removed from life, the simplest of tasks seem immeasurably complicated, experiences that would usually bring you joy are marred by the constant nagging of your exhaustion ('I would be enjoying myself so much more if I weren't so tired!'). You start looking at other people and wishing you were them, whoever they are and whatever they are doing, just because they appear more rested than you. You watch a television programme and the scenes of couples dozing in bed or even children tucked in for the night about to embark on an interruption-free night fill you with jealousy, even though you know they are actors and it's all fiction. Your body and brain are begging you to sleep, and nothing else matters.

We find ourselves in these situations usually because something has happened in our life that is making sleep impossible. It might be illness (yours or someone close), or it might be something subtler, such as a worry gnawing at you (though you may not be consciously aware of what that worry is), or it might be pregnancy, and in a lot of cases, small children and babies. Whatever it is that is challenging your sleep is most likely not something you can readily change. Indeed, trying to 'change' anything – i.e. fix it – can contribute to your feelings of exhaustion and of being 'trapped' in a sleep-deprived state.

When we had our first baby, we didn't get much sleep at all. A difficult birth, a colicky baby, new-parent anxiety, a longing for our old lives to please come back, fear of doing the 'wrong thing'. We were walking zombies, exhausted and yet unable to sleep. During this time, we obsessively researched ways to fix the problem – the problem obviously being the baby and not us. Any new parent will know that there is a phenomenal amount of material available online and elsewhere offering advice and practical suggestions for getting your child to sleep more during the night. If you read through enough of it, the advice soon starts to contradict itself (feed your baby more, feed them less, make sure they sleep in pitch black, make sure they have a little nightlight on, put them to bed earlier, put them to bed later, etc.). A rational look at all the information soon makes it clear that most people have no idea how to get babies to sleep better at night, but that eventually, most babies do end up sleeping well enough at some point, before too long. However, lost in new-parent anxiety and sleep deprivation, we implemented a number of the suggested strategies, all the while worrying whether we were doing them 'right', then becoming consumed by that worry, and then worrying again about our sleep-lessness, and then not surprisingly worrying even more as we witnessed each 'solution' to have very little effect on our baby's sleep. We became even more obsessed with our own lack of sleep. The less able we felt ourselves of fixing the sleep problem, the more we felt its impact, the more we worried about its impact, the more tired we became, the more we longed for our baby to sleep more, the more solutions we sought to fix the problem. . .

We immersed ourselves in the problem, worried about the problem never going away, tried to work out why the problem was there in the first place, wondered if we were making the problem worse or better. We lay in bed wide-awake, thinking of ways to ensure we would get a good night's sleep. This says it all.

What we didn't do was stop. We didn't consider that the best course of action was to do nothing, and as much of nothing as possible. We didn't consider that rather than spending hours reading about baby sleep patterns or staying up late whenever we had got the baby to sleep at a half-decent hour to 'enjoy' some time off from trying to get the baby to sleep, we should down tools, relax and perhaps even enjoy the hazy, fuzzy feeling of tiredness and use it as an excuse – a reason – to take things slow and hang about in our pyjamas as often as possible, to stare into space, to be excused from doing, or to allow ourselves the excuse of not doing anything that well. We didn't consider the possibility that it was OK to be tired for a few months, or that it was perfectly normal. We didn't trust that things would shift and soon enough we all would be sleeping for hours again.

It's very easy to talk wisely about such difficult periods in life when they are over, but we faced it all over again when we had a second child and managed the situation (by not trying to manage it) far better. We accepted that our best line of attack was accept-ance: of the baby's likely unfavourable sleep habits, and that we would be tired. While one of us tended to the baby, the other slept. If we had a hard night, we cancelled plans for the next day. We let our oldest child watch more TV than usual. We snuggled. We stared into the abyss. We allowed our tiredness to be there, and as a result, it didn't feel so heavy or so serious, and soon enough, it lifted (and then came back again. . . and went. . . and, well, we're still going through it).

Without obsessing over sleep and instead merely accepting that tiredness was something we were going to experience for a while, we didn't feel exhausted all the time (though there certainly were and are still days during which we feel completely exhausted, but this is life). Most notably, by worrying less about how any of us sleeps, the sleep that we do get is more restful and comes more easily.

What happens when we do sleep?

There is still a lot to learn about sleep. For instance, although it is possible to monitor brains in different sleep states, scientists are still unclear as to how to promote more (or less) of certain stages of sleep. What science is certain of is that the right balance of all the sleep states is what leaves us feeling rested and well. It is therefore useful to understand the different stages of sleep, as we currently know them, and if you plan on taking a nap to understand how long to go for in order to be left feeling refreshed rather than befuddled.

PRE-SLEEP: When you go to sleep, you pass through a pre-sleep stage. Your body might jerk itself awake at this point (although technically, you are still awake) and you might see imagery and have a waking dream. James often shouts out during this state, proclaiming such things as, 'I'm flying in a space burger!' and 'I think it's some kind of custard!'. Clearly, it can be quite a strange and pleasant experience.

STAGES ONE AND TWO: As sleep begins to seduce you, your body falls into the first two stages of sleep. They are distinct in what happens to the body and brain but, to keep it simple, they are similar in terms of their outcome. Both lead us to feeling refreshed, to a lesser (stage one) or greater (stage two) degree.

Typically, in the first stage (the first few minutes after pre-sleep) we experience an increase in creativity and problem solving, so if we wake up from here we're brighter and more refreshed in our thinking. Then comes stage two, which typically takes up to 20 minutes after entering the pre-sleep stage. If we wake up or are woken up from here, it takes perhaps a few minutes to come fully back online, but it leaves us feeling refreshed, our mood is elevated and we're more energised and less sleepy.

DEEP: After around 20 minutes, we can cross the chasm into deep sleep. This is the tricky bit: it's very good for our body, it's hard to control and you'll feel very groggy if you're suddenly woken from it. Typically, it's hard to rouse people from deep sleep, and if we do, we might get a grumpy checked-out person in the room. It'll likely take them a while to come around (they're experiencing what we call 'sleep inertia'). This helps us to see why a 10–20-minute nap can leave us feeling perky but a 40-minute snooze dazed and confused.

When you go to sleep at night, you cycle around (not literally) every 90 minutes from light to deep to dream sleep, and then back to waking up. Each night, you'll have lots of these waking moments, though you probably won't notice them. Deeper sleep tends to come in the first two or three cycles of the night, and then we slip into more dream sleep as the night progresses. For a while, it was believed that deep sleep was the most essential component of a good night's rest, rather than a winning combination of all stages.

With this basic understanding of sleep, you might already see why you sometimes wake up feeling alert and ready-to-go, and other times as though you want to go straight back to bed. If you can, you might even see how altering your sleep schedule – shifting your alarm, going to bed a little later or earlier – might aid a good night's sleep.

Although it might be hard to plan your whole night around these stages (especially if you are being woken up by factors outside of your control), at least understanding them might help you see that it's not always the amount of sleep that you are getting, but the process and stages of sleep experienced that affect how you feel. A short nap can be more refreshing than a long nap – that's a pretty sizable discovery if you want to catch some extra sleep but fear you don't have time.

There are always exceptions to these rules, of course. Some people find they can't snooze at all without feeling groggy, while others seem immune to the effects of sleep inertia, able to nap anytime, any place, and feel refreshed regardless of how long they've slept. Some people go crashing into deep sleep within moments of falling asleep, others scrape by with only minutes of deep sleep cobbled together some time just before dawn. Some of us need only four of these cycles to wake up feeling refreshed, others need six. Science is still in debate about the concept of 'sleep debt' – whether or not sleep can be banked and credited. All we know is that all of us need *enough* sleep, and enough is only measurable by you.

It's 4am and you've woken up and can't get back to sleep. Or, perhaps it's midnight and sleep is yet to arrive at your door. There could be a whole variety of reasons this has happened. Maybe you had too much stimulus before bedtime, or not enough time and space to be with the events of the day. Rather than trying to work out 'why' or getting frustrated at your failings to get yourself off to sleep, how would it be to embrace what's going on?

If we start to resist our restlessness, it's likely to continue. We feel restless about feeling restless and our mind begins to tell stories such as, 'I'll never get to sleep' or 'I'm going to feel so tired in the morning!'. These fears and concerns about our inability to sleep are quite natural, but we are fighting our experience and trying to get away from what's happening and away from ourselves. It's not very restful.

If, however, we can make a generous space for our restlessness, then there's the potential for everything to change. When we give up the struggle and fall into our wakeful experience wherever and whenever it might be, we have the opportunity to meet a naturally occurring 'close-to-sleep' phenomenon that creates a shift in our brain chemistry, which is a wonderful gift and antidote to our restlessness.

When we rest close to the edge of sleep, the two sides of that edge might fuse into a 'waking dream' state, when we are neither awake nor asleep. This is your opportunity to practise it:

- As you find yourself unable to sleep, or get back to sleep, rather than fight the experience, can you embrace it? Consider this time as an opportunity to be with yourself, and rest

- Engage with what you've learned from other practice experiments in this book: find a restful position, settle in and, if helpful, follow your breath, observe the spaces between breaths or pay attention to bodily sensations or the feeling of your body in relationship with the surfaces and space that surround it

- Allow your mind to shift from worry about the lack of sleep to a looser, more accepting state

- Begin to notice what rises up in the mind as abstract images or new feelings and sensations, or even what you might hear in your inner voice

- Give up trying to 'work anything out' and instead listen fully to your experience

- Let yourself drift here. It's quite natural to move between the analytical mind (over-thinking) and this in-between state

Paying attention to your natural rhythms

As with most things in life, we all have our own peculiarities, predilections and natural tendencies. Sleep is no different. How you sleep is affected by external factors, your inherent programming and your preferences.

For millennia, human beings rested and became active to the rhythm of the sun. In that way, light has a significant effect on us. For this reason, technology – from the basic (household lighting) to the more advanced (smartphones and tablets) – can disturb our natural cues for sleep. How we interact with nature can also affect our body's ability to recognise when it's time to sleep and when it's time to 'work'. If you don't get outside in daylight during the winter, you're likely to feel the urge to hibernate and feel lethargic (and possibly even low). Your biology is telling you it's sleep-time because it can't see any light. In contrast, if your bedtime routine involves brushing your teeth under the glare of a fluorescent light, then you might find yourself unexpectedly wired as your head hits the pillow – your body is thinking 'Morning!'.

In addition to this, we each have our own unique biological preferences for waking and sleeping. Some of us are naturally early risers, whereas others are not ready to be roused much before 10am. This has nothing to do with laziness or rebelliousness, but our inherent makeup, as well as our age (teenagers need more sleep and tend to operate on a later schedule). Society's insistence on starting early is desperately out of synch with some people's natural cycles. It might be helpful – or a relief – to consider that your tiredness might not be your fault.

It is possible to influence your natural rhythms, however, and perhaps this is good news if you're a natural night owl with a young family and nine-to-five job. This must be done slowly over time, little by little, though always remember that left to its own devices, your body will fall back into its natural pattern. As always, be gentle, kind and forgiving.

Observing what might be your natural sleep preferences can ease a lot of the shame and labelling around them. For example, either being a late riser or party pooper. When you know your rhythm, you can either adjust it to adapt to life, or relax back in to knowing that your programming is perfect and natural.

ASK YOURSELF

If you had no commitments, what would be your preferred time to go to bed? What would be your preferred time to get up in the morning? When do you feel most energised/able to get on with tasks? When do you tend to want to down tools and do nothing? Similarly, have you noticed whether taking a nap in the day leaves you feeling more energised, or less? Does this change depending on when you nap?

How much can we control our sleep?

We've already used the term 'sleep hygiene' and it has become a popular means to describe the steps we can take to help us fall asleep and sleep better. There's no harm in following such advice, but always remember that if it doesn't work, it doesn't mean you're necessarily doing anything wrong. Let's not make sleep another thing we can be failing at. Sleep, as we have established, remains at some levels, mysterious. Our experience is that some of the sleep hygiene recommendations make a difference, and some don't. It should also be remembered that for most people, their sleep habits are not entirely theirs to own anyway, with small people dictating when and for how long they sleep or partners in the bed next to them operating to their own sleep patterns, and all the other outside distractions of neighbours coming and going, the early morning postman, traffic in the road. . . We don't want to start worrying about sleep hygiene as well as sleep.

The first thing we are encouraged to consider is that the time before bed and the time in the morning when you wake up should be all about preparing for and recovering from sleep. We should expect and make allowances for the fact that we are likely to feel groggy on waking (perhaps we can enjoy this 'quiet' time rather than bemoan or begrudge it). In the same way that it's not a good idea to send messages or make phone calls when you're drunk, it's not a good idea to rely too much on your early morning cognitions. Although, having said that, there might be moments of insight that we access upon waking. This is a natural part of waking up and it's a good idea to write them down or note them in some way so that you can come back to them later (notice these insights didn't come from you 'figuring anything out,' so don't try to figure them out now). Celebrate the sleepy-ness of the morning. Gaze out the window. Take your time to make breakfast. Have a leisurely shower. Allow any feelings of grogginess to be there. Do everything you can to allow for a restful morning, even if that means preparing for the day the night before.

And about the night before: we all want to wind down at night, usually we're tired, but perhaps we ought to pay a little more attention to how we're choosing to spend the last couple hours before bed. We've already suggested that, for some of us, the things we think are restful do not always leave us feeling rested, and in that way, the things we think might be helping us to wind down at night might be winding us up. Annoyingly, the things so many of us love to do to relax in the evening might be having the opposite effect: watching television, having a glass of wine and a nibble of chocolate, scrolling through our social media feeds. These activities might actually be stimulating your system – the sugar and caffeine in the chocolate, the light from your screens and your emotional response to what you're viewing. It could be worth cutting some out or moving them to earlier in the day and seeing what happens. Perhaps approach the last hour-and-a-half of the day as though it were your first sleep cycle. Keep it dark and snugly. Read a book. Listen to some relaxing music or podcast. Find out what works for you.

Regardless of the science, what do you observe?

We felt it important to give you a basic understanding of sleep, but we also wanted to return to some elements of our previous messages: ones that help you unwind, let go, feel at ease and find a sense of peace that's already here. It's important to recognise that while science is a very important tool in helping us to better understand ourselves and the nature of the human body, it cannot replace or even over-rule our direct experience. Ultimately, we have to become our own scientists, so we'd like to propose, again, that you approach any and all of the ideas presented above with a degree of scrutiny.

ASK YOURSELF

What helps you get the best night's sleep? Experiment and see what, if anything, makes a difference. Switch off your phone at 8pm for a couple of nights; scroll through your favourite social media feed until your head hits the pillow the next. You might find that eating chocolate and watching a slushy movie might be the very things that help you to sleep – the endorphin hit from eating chocolate can easily off-set its stimulatory effects. Checking your phone might give you peace of mind rather than worry, and watching your favourite TV show can make you laugh yourself into feeling relaxed and give you a sense of coming together with your family or loved ones. No one can tell you what will work for you.

Some sleep experts suggest we should all remove our televisions from our houses and spend our evenings talking and sharing the events of our day. We can only say how stressful that would be for us in our house. We love watching movies, and it's hilarious to observe our little children bobbing up and down to the theme of their favourite programme. It gives us a few moments' respite from building dens and answering endless questions about e.g. the death of next door's goldfish. We've never noticed a correlation between our kids' sleep and their TV habits.

Think about these suggestions for helping you sleep as a set of enquiries to experiment with. Stay light with it and see what might bring you ease, peace and relaxation. All you can do is try to observe. You might be a natural rule breaker, and good for you.

If you give yourself over entirely to science, you are at its whim. It's not uncommon for 'proven' scientific theories to later be super-seded or built upon. It's also true that how we feel about something cannot be the only measure of things. Our preconceptions and beliefs (we all have them, whether we see them or not) mean that we must check our references with friends, loved ones and family, but, likewise, when those close to us tell us we are a certain way, we should also take that with a pinch of salt. None of us sees clearly.

That sleep is such a popular subject today might have you believe it's a new 'problem'. It might be more of an issue, perhaps, but methods for feeling better rested and sleeping deeper have been written down and shared for thousands of years, and these are constantly re-introduced and written in ever-new language to appeal to the culture of the time. So even thousands of years ago, when people were apparently less frantic and distracted, sleep was still a conundrum for many. Don't believe the hype.

But don't not believe it either.

Rest, regardless of sleep

When we become aware of our natural sleep patterns and understand what happens during sleep and appreciate what might be affecting the quality of our sleep, we are equipped to understand our feelings of tiredness, lethargy and perhaps even our unease.

We'd like to bring you back to the core message of this book: that there is part of you that is untouched and untainted by anything, including sleep. Whether you've had enough, too much or too little, the 'no-thing' that you inhabit when you are nowhere else, is utterly untouched. To lean into this knowledge (this awareness, to be more accurate) at times when we're feeling especially tired can offer great relief.

Just as we rest less during the times we need rest the most, we often sleep least when we need it the most: when we're worried, when we're busy, and of course, when we're parenting young children. At the time you most need tolerance, patience and forbearance, our sleep-deprived brains are at their worst in terms of dealing with the toddler who doesn't yet understand that mummy and daddy are just tired that day, and that they need to give us a break. The executive who needs all their resources to strategise and find creative new ways to work with challenging problems is least likely to be able to do this when they are tired, stressed and undernourished. In exploring some of the practical suggestions here, it could also be that the simple practice of resting back into your wholeness (that is already and always within you) is the one and only resource you have in such challenging times.

This is where the practice of 'restful being' comes to life for us. In the midst of our most difficult circumstances, can we lean back into that part of us that is already OK. We find our centre (which is indeed centreless and cannot be found. . .). We can feel the openness of our consciousness that is already balanced, healthy, healed and deeply at ease amidst circumstances that are quite the contrary. We might be heavy with exhaustion, but we can be refreshed by the experience of stepping beyond our tiredness and witnessing the lightness of being that pervades all our experience.

Enquiry 17:
What happens when you wake up slowly?

It's 4 a.m. and you find yourself waking up, for no apparent reason. You have the option here to try to get back to sleep (see Enquiry 16, page 209) or to explore the freshness and openness of this early waking state. This is the other 'edge' of that between-sleep experience we talked about. It is called the hypnopompic state and it's one of the most profound ways to realise the state that we constantly address in this book; to find that which lies beyond the thinking mind and sense of self.

When we wake, it takes some time for our thinking mind to come 'online'. This can be a challenge if you have to leap in to action, or a great gift if you have the time to explore it:

- *On waking, resist the temptation to immediately move, shift position or engage with your physical body*

- *Even if you do find yourself moving, begin to observe the feeling or state that you find yourself in. Let labels like 'sleepy' or 'confused' fall away and simply rest into it*

- *If the mind begins to churn, let it be there, but notice that there's a natural perspective from thoughts. That you can watch them come and go within this 'sleepiness' or spaciousness*

- *Explore the location of this feeling of spaciousness. Where does it begin? Where does it end? Does this feel familiar to you? Have you known this state before?*

If you're not a person who wakes in the middle of the night, it may seem that your life doesn't provide the opportunity to wake up slowly in this way. However, there's plenty of opportunity to do this if you want to. If, for example, you wake up to an alarm each morning, you can set yourself up to 'wake up gently' by setting the alarm for 20 minutes (or even 10 minutes) earlier. If your habit is to wake up and 'hit' the snooze button, see if you can do so slowly, with a quality of ease and gentleness, and then slip back under the covers and explore this state. Follow the prompts above. Have fun!

All The Rest

So, you are resting more, or seeing how you were already resting throughout your waking life and noticing these moments, allowing them, lingering in the echoes of the experience. You're living life knowing that your downtime is as valuable as your uptime. You've learnt to stop trying to stop and instead just stop. You are the hamster who has jumped off the wheel and is, at last, making progress – a new kind of progress that's more like an evolution, a becoming that feels effortless and entirely yours. You are winning! You've softened, you've taken yourself in, given yourself a hug (bear, or straight up snuggle) and told yourself that, actually, amid the chaos and turbulence of this life of yours, beneath and beyond it all, you are perfect. You are, in fact, more than perfect.

— *You are the space in which perfection can appear.*

You are everything, and nothing. You are that which sits between the opposites. You are that which is neither awake nor asleep. You are that moment between each breath, not breathing in and not breathing out. You are the awareness that we all feel when everything else is gone. You are everywhere and nowhere. You *are*, and that is enough – it is amazing.

And yet you still have to buy toilet roll.

This is the problem a lot of us have after our great awakenings. We see the blissful truth of our existence and, bar perhaps a few weeks or days of walking on air, we find our lives on a day-to-day basis to be the same. We have the same family, the same friends, the same house, the same weird collection of stuff in that catchall drawer where we put old and new batteries and never know which is which, the 52 bus is still the 52 bus and there's always that one odd man who sits at the back breathing heavily, and then there are still the holidays that don't go the way we'd imagined and those nights out that gave us no more joy than if we'd stayed in and watched reruns of that old sitcom from the Nineties that for some reason is just so cosy-making, and we still find ourselves losing the remote control even though we've established a dedicated place for it, and leave the fridge full of half-full/empty jars of chutney and that last hunk of parmesan cheese that somehow is still not quite green.

So, what is the point of any of this if life does not *change*?

If you are already, at your essence, everything you have ever wanted and are ever possible of being, then awakenings are nothing more than a moment – or collection of moments – in which you realise that fact. They are not the fact themselves. For this reason, between 'awakenings', you might not feel any different in a way that is always apparent. That is to say: when you rest, in the way we have described in this book, you might at times feel amazing as a result, and there will also be times when you don't feel any different to how you felt before reading this book. We have not written a prescription for a great new life. Instead, we hope to have offered you a new perspective from which to see yourself and your place in existence, and as a result feel a newfound sense of peace with who you are and what's happening around you. This will not likely cause a sudden catapulting into a new state of being but more a gentle and continuous stepping into an awareness that, albeit subtle, is unyielding, reassuring and real.

Life may not change, but your relationship with it will. With rest on your agenda of things to not-do, as you recognise more and more glimpses of that all-pervading unshakable awareness that is the essence of who you are, and as you accept that the future holds no better version of you than is here already, you will engage with life with a newfound sense of lightness and ease.

Learning to 'be' is an up and down process; the outcome of it is invariably to feel more relaxed, more at ease with where and who we are, and we cannot pretend we don't desire this outcome. As much as we know it is contrary to rest, we will start *trying* to rest. We still start *trying* to stop. We will start trying to control our rest. . . and we will feel restless as a result.

This will happen, and we can be OK with this happening. Whenever you feel unease, whenever you realise you are trying to find rest, don't fight it or berate yourself. Welcome your restlessness. Have a little giggle at it. Be easy on yourself.

'Welcome unease with ease' might be the simplest way to sum up everything in this book.

Rest, effort and ease

We hope you have absorbed that we are not advocates of stopping everything all the time – that you can both 'be' and 'do', and in fact this is balance, and this is life.

But there is an interesting enquiry to be had when we consider our relationship with effort, and then consider what happens when effort becomes stress. Or the opposite: when taking time out might slip into detachment, or even despondency.

As we have explored, effort and any associated pain or stress from that effort is not something that is measurable in a universal capacity, but is it possible that there might be some kind of 'restful effort'?

If we take physical exercise as a simple example of effort, we can consider the point at which our exertion starts to feel more than a little uncomfortable – when we are perhaps even suffering. Exactly when we reach this stage varies for all of us, but it might be worth considering whether at this point you drive yourself to push through, or see it as a signpost to ease off, and then how your decision leaves you feeling (physically and emotionally). Only you are able to decipher where your point of having pushed too far is, and you can only discover this by listening to yourself. No one can tell you that you were wrong to give up, or right to stop.

Our relationships might be another area where we consider what the 'right amount' of effort to put in is. We accept that life with another person will inevitably involve compromises, unpleasant discoveries, aspects of ourselves being reflected back to us that we do not like, etc., but the overall expectation is that the stress of the effort will be outweighed by the benefits of having someone (someone in particular) by your side. But only you know when your relationship has gone beyond the point of 'constructive effort' (or whatever you wish to call it), and very often this comes as a sense of just knowing, that is beyond knowledge (or 'your truth').

ASK YOURSELF

Can you think of any aspect of your life right now where you might be exhausting yourself (emotionally or physically) through effort?

We can't tell you where your personal point of 'gone-too-far' is when it comes to any aspect of your life, but we can promise that, for example, it is possible to be healthy and fit without punishing yourself. In fact, you are more likely to fall into being fit and healthy if you approach yourself with inquisitive kindness – being with yourself, listening to yourself, sensing into your body and becoming aware of how it is feeling. We so rarely look at ourselves without judgement, and so how can we really know who we are and what we might need?

We will always have things to do – things that we have to do, things that we want to do and things that we're not too fussed about one way or another. As we rest and allow ourselves to do nothing, to relinquish control, to welcome experience just as it presents itself to us, we find ourselves tapping into that underlying ease – that open awareness that is already here, already the case, always. As this happens, we find all aspects of life have the potential to exist in front of a backdrop of ease. That is, the ease that seemed so far away now feels closer (and if it doesn't, we know how to remind ourselves that it is). We might drive ourselves, we might work hard to develop a fitter body or maintain our relationship, but we do so knowing that beyond it all, we are held by an unending well of stillness that is here now, and will be here whether we have achieved the things we set out to achieve by our efforts, or not.

Can I use medication to help me rest?

We would never advocate giving up any medication you may have been prescribed. Sleeping pills, for example, can take you to the land of nod, and although we know (because science tells us) that you are unlikely to get the ratio of deep, light and REM sleep that will lead to you feeling as rested as you would had you taken yourself there yourself, they might be just the thing to break a vicious cycle. Similarly, for some people, antidepressants will see them through a difficult patch in the way they otherwise might not have managed, offering just enough buoyancy for them to start exploring what else they might do (or not do!) to help navigate back to dry land.

We're big fans of medicine and science. Scientists help us to understand the world; medicines help us to heal our bodies. There are mistakes, imperfections, wrong conclusions – all the things that come with being human, of course – but today we have at our disposal remarkable treatments and mind-blowing technologies that allow us to understand our bodies and minds in incredibly useful and insightful ways. The best thing you can do for yourself is open your mind to it all. Keep informed and keep aware, inside and out.

Right now, there are storms brewing, the is sun shining, rivers are drying up, homes flooding, crops thriving, villages starving, empires building, economies collapsing, babies being born, families fighting, music being composed, murders plotted, cakes baking and lions sinking their teeth into the raw flesh of another beast, and somewhere you are reading a book about rest.

The world is happening, and you are happening within that happening. For as long as you are alive, this is not going to change. There will be happenings you want to be involved in, others you don't; happenings you want to change, others you don't notice. This is life.

There will always be aspects of your life that you wish to alter, change, move around, move through and seek relief from. You will always have obstacles to overcome, experiences to learn from, new people to meet, people to let go, insights to come, surprises, treats, moments of inexplicable clarity and moments of inexplicable confusion, grief and panic. None of us lives a life without challenge, change or chaos. We are all vulnerable to the unpredictable unfolding of life. Maybe it's a great big mess, maybe it's a masterfully orchestrated cosmic happening of significant meaning and purpose. We do not know. You do not know. Whatever, there is a backdrop to this happening that remains aware, constant and unbreakable. You have already glimpsed this awareness, and the more you notice these glimpses, and the more you allow these glimpses to happen to you, the

228

more you are able to find relief in knowing your awareness is always there and always OK – even when your life circumstances are far, far from OK.

When you recognise the importance of stepping back from all the happenings to see what lies beyond it all, the happenings become clearer. You can see how you fit among them, how you can influence them, and how you can't. And you know that when the happenings overwhelm you, you can stop, and rest.

As you begin to see yourself more clearly and recognise that while you experience feelings, sensations and thoughts, you are not any of these things, you will start to see the world in the same way – not bound by how you see or think about it, and, ultimately, no different from you.

There will always be challenges, worries, annoying relatives, dishes in the sink, bad weather, global disasters, bizarre election results, ant infestations and nothing on the TV. We all consider ourselves to have problems, and we each feel the significance of these problems very differently. Different things affect each of us differently at different times in our lives and even at different times in our day, and we will never entirely know why. All we can do is review the data, do what feels right, and let it all go.

Even in times of extreme tragedy, we can find relief – even if only marginally – in exploring what it might be like to *be* with our emotions without trying to understand, work through or do anything with or about them at all. As we detach conditions, expectations and desire from our feelings, we might glimpse the space that holds them – a space that remains shatterproof even when the most distressing of events unfold. A space in which we are always inhabiting, that is always us.

Behind the whirling, tiring, confusing chaos of life is a backdrop of stillness. It is everything. It is nothing. It is you.

The journey home

It's our hope, that as you've taken this journey of doing nothing, of 'giving up' (and then giving up the giving up), of going beyond knowing and of having and of letting go of any desire for an outcome or destination, that you have had, however fleeting, a moment (or moments) of insight.

There may have been points along the way when you felt a clarity dawning or emotion breaking through. The relief of understanding or experiencing ourselves as already whole, already complete, can be tremendous. We might feel moved. We might feel this truth in our hearts. We might *feel* our hearts for the first time in a long time, or indeed forever.

(We might not.)

You may have wept for the disowned parts of yourself, those that you put off for the future or claimed to be in your past and felt ashamed of. (You may have laughed.) As these aspects of our self and our mind fall away, we get more of that true self shining through, and its arrival is often heralded by a sense of relief, or a feeling of falling back in love with where we are and who we are, just as we are.

In the years that we have been sharing these teachings we've met many people from different walks of life – from the wealthy to the less well-off, bright-minded intellectuals to the sensitive 'feelers' of life, those from the East and those from the West, the old and the young – and there is a common theme for everyone: that after taking this journey with us they experience an unmistakable sense of coming home.

— *When we rest, we are in our sanctuary, and it is entirely of our own being.*

Our restful sanctuary will never need a new roof, it is never locked and it will never be anywhere but within us. Nothing outside of our own being can alter this fact. Nothing outside of our own being can alter who we really are, and we are always, entirely, wholly in love with ourselves, whatever we have done, wish to do or have had done against us.

When all is said and done, we are all in search of love. Not the conditional kind of love that tires over time, but the unconditioned embrace of a truer self that has never wanted anything of you and never had conditions and has never been in conflict with or resisted anything you have ever experienced. This love embraces you (and everything else) just as you are.

In any moments in which you have felt moved or experienced a sudden sweeping ease or a physical shift in your body, a relaxation in the breath or an insight about feeling somehow whole again, these are signs of that self shining through. That knowing coming back to itself. That sense of returning to something familiar and deeply comforting. The 'you' that is beyond description, measure or qualification. That 'you' who you know is your truth, your completeness, your unshakable restful being.

Welcome home.

Rest in Times of Crisis

This is a new chapter in *The Book of Rest* and we're writing it in the middle of a global health crisis. A pandemic is sweeping country after country. In the UK, we've just come out of three months of national lockdown, whereby we were not to leave our homes unless to take limited exercise or buy essentials such as groceries and medicine. All public spaces, non-essential shops and leisure facilities were closed. Schools remained open only to children whose parents worked in industries and services deemed critical. All other employees were either furloughed or instructed to work at home, and if you had school-age children it became your responsibility to help them undertake their studies.

These restrictions were applied to everyone: the rich, the poor, the famous, the anonymous and everyone in between. Social media stopped being a platform on which to share images of glamorous nights out, exotic holidays or the signature dish at that exclusive eatery. Everyone was stuck at home. Television production was halted. Blockbuster movies had nowhere to be shown, so they went straight to the small screen. All shows, music, festivals and public events stopped. There were no planes in the sky, the roads were empty, city centres were deserted and business parks became like ghost towns.

— The trappings of our existence were removed.

The terror and relief of change

For some, these changes brought surprising relief. Working from home meant no stressful commute and more time for family. With a ban on leaving the house, the pressure was off to seek adventure and experiences beyond those available in your back yard. With little to spend on travel, no option to buy meals or drinks out and certainly no holidays or weekends away, the cost of living went down. Communities came together to offer support and inspiration. Windows were decorated with rainbows. Many people recounted that they had rediscovered the joys of a simple life and seen how many of the things they'd deemed essential for a happy and fulfilling existence were not missed when gone. For them, fewer choices did not equate to lesser experiences. They took solace in nature and appreciated the new quiet that permeated even the heart of the city – cities that now were no longer shrouded in smog. You could see the sky. The air was fresher. Pleasures, it seemed, could come for free, without leaving home or spending money or indeed *having* anything new. For some, lockdown was a balm revealing unexpected treasures. Joy was experienced not by achievement or acquisition, but by subtraction. Delight could be found in the slow, the simple, the already-there.

— But this is not the full picture.

In addition to the threat and consequences of falling ill, the pandemic has presented a host of further challenges and hardships. With national lockdown, many lost their jobs, businesses folded, domestic violence increased and healthcare became seemingly inaccessible. This time of restriction and uncertainty has put a huge strain on our mental health. Fear is a hungry beast and it takes a hardy constitution not to be dragged into its lair.

The year 2020 has brought both worry and respite. Indeed, a palpable theme of the pandemic has been our propensity to experience extreme opposites in emotions. One minute we're rejoicing at having more time to spend with our children, the next we're desperate for space. One day we're feeling productive and healthy, the next we're hitting the chocolate stash and wasting hours scrolling online. We yo-yo between welcoming change in our world ('the planet is healing', 'we won't take anything for granted ever again') to panicking about what kind of a future awaits us and our children ('will things ever be normal again?'). We have never been here before, so we have no way to navigate any of it. It's dizzying.

This time has also made especially evident great polarities in our interpretation of the world around us. We might focus on how a global health crisis can unite humankind as we come together to fight a common threat. Alternatively, we can see how that same threat causes distrust, disruption and friction as we negotiate an appropriate response.

The pandemic has not been the only globally transformative event of the year. In May 2020, George Floyd, a 46-year-old African-American, died as the result of injuries sustained during his arrest by a white police officer. Protests took place around the world, led by the Black Lives Matter movement, and leading figures in politics, media, entertainment and sport pledged to combat systemic racism. Historical figures celebrated in the names of organisations, buildings and streets were brought into question for their associations with the black slave trade, and their statues were torn down without debate. Not only was our future in question, but the past was brought under scrutiny.

In the UK, there was the looming deadline for Britain's exit from the European Union and the changes that would bring. In 2020, whatever you thought of them, it became clear that the structures of our society were not set in stone.

The truth about our existence

When we finished writing the first edition of this book, we had no idea how pertinent its contents would be just a few months after its publication; that the concept of being able to find calm within yourself amidst a chaotic world outside would become relevant to *most* people. We also had no idea the extent to which personally the events of 2020 would compel us to practise what we preach. Like most people, our work, home and relationship were forced into new frameworks, and the things we had planned and relied on were gone. We had to rethink and rearrange everything, and do so with a focus only on the immediate future. Any long-term planning was a matter of extreme guesswork. At times, it felt like we had been placed in a pressure cooker, and with a ban on leaving the house, there was no escape.

What 2020 has revealed is not so much that we are vulnerable, but more that the structures in which we arrange our lives are. If ever there was a time to seek out the unyielding steadiness of your internal world against the ever-changing and unreliable arrangement of the external world, it is now.

Why is rest so important in times of crisis?

Resting is a process of surrender; of allowing yourself to be released from the trappings of your desires, your circumstances, your preferences, your beliefs. Your deepest awareness asks no questions and needs no answers, but to fall into this freest aspect of yourself you have to relinquish your longing to have everything figured out.

This is easier to do when life feels easy and safe. When you have a regular income and your children are being educated and taken care of in school, when you have easy access to food and essentials and no barriers to being with family and friends, when you don't feel your physical wellbeing is under particular threat, it's easier to trust in life. We feel less of a pull towards control and order (because things seem fairly controlled and ordered) and the thought of stopping, releasing into that place where we have no influence and no direction (where we are only *being*), is less daunting.

When we're afraid, or confused, or conflicted, we seek answers, assurance, certainties. Something to give us a sense of steadiness. Something outside of ourselves to make us feel better. We seek an *external* anchor.

But the challenge with seeking such a thing in times of crisis is that there are very few such anchors to be found.

— Rest is a doorway to your internal anchor – one that can always be found and remains accessible regardless of external events.

When we allow ourselves to stop and fall into deep rest, we experience the part of ourselves that remains steady even in the most turbulent of times. This is vital to our maintaining a sense of calm, and without it, a crisis – personal or global – can leave us feeling overwhelmed and anxious. Making a point of seeking out rest – of deliberately allowing ourselves a moment to slip into that spacious nowhere, which is the backdrop to all our experiences – can be a lifeline. This need not be a dedicated meditation practice or anything more than taking a twenty-minute lie-down away from all distractions and devices. It might even just be a commitment to not picking up your smartphone so often, or to loiter in a mid-morning gaze out the window. The beauty is that such seemingly small gestures can have an enormous impact on your overall wellbeing.

Lockdown provided a rare opportunity to float in the unknown and experience ourselves without the distraction of routines or being anywhere other than alone, at home. Our place within the world was made less distinct. The pressure to be doing great or impressive things was eased. We were given a freedom, of sorts. However, our resistance, as humans seeking order, to this opportunity became palpable on social media as we scrambled to share our quarantine achievements: a revamped garden, a kitchen makeover, the fruition of weeks and weeks of craft projects. The desire to be seen to be productive and resourceful won over the opportunity to release, retreat and rest.

When everything around you seems to be falling apart, it's hard to trust that you are not also breaking into pieces. Any semblance of feeling steady and safe might feel like it's slipping further from your reach. We would propose, however, that just as the events of 2020 offered some the opportunity to realise that we don't need particular things and experiences to feel fulfilled, we now also have the opportunity to see that we do not need an ordered external world to experience the steady sanctuary of our innate wellbeing.

How to approach rest in turbulent times

Just as it shuttles the practical makeup of our lives into unfamiliar territory, crises such as a pandemic will, to a lesser or greater extent, shake us up psychologically.

There are few people resilient to the nature of a global emergency. Therefore, the first thing to do is to recognise any feelings of being unsettled – of being restless or even sleepless – are not a sign that there is anything wrong with you. It's a natural and normal reaction, and your body (and being) will thank you for acknowledging its entitlement to be out of sorts.

Of course, you don't want to feel restless and on edge forever. So, the next step, once you have allowed yourself to feel what you are feeling, is to explore these feelings from a different, deeper perspective – to take a step back from them and see how they are not rigid or as powerful as you might have first thought them to be.

Even with less extreme events and changes in our lives, we all dance between feeling in control and then, as the illusion is shattered, vulnerable. We bounce between these extreme positions, while the truth lies beyond them. The nature of our deepest being is able to watch these two extremes without preference, knowing that neither one is 'real'.

What do you notice when you take a moment to welcome in change? How does your body feel? Does the idea of change leave you feeling light, bubbly and effervescent, or contracted, rigid and scared? Or something else? If you take a moment to honour these 'communications', consider what they might be showing you about yourself. Don't seek out a definite answer, just ask the question and wait and see.

For most of us, change brings two apparently opposing feelings: resistance and excitement. It's rare to feel excitement without also experiencing nerves. Similarly, as much as we crave adventure and novelty, we seek out the familiar and comfortable. These opposites endlessly play out with each other throughout our entire life (sometimes at precisely the same time, as we will for things to stay the same and change all at once).

By recognising both these 'faces of change' we are less likely to get stuck in one or the other, and we're likely to feel less afraid of being out of control. If we can give a bit of space and mental airtime to both of these 'urges', they might equalise one another and leave us feeling more spacious within ourselves, freer and open to all possibilities.

Discovering a place where there is no uncertainty

Uncertainty can both excite and unnerve us, but there is always a deeper part of us that has no investment in the details and events of our lives being one way or another. As we become more familiar with this aspect of ourselves, we find a stability to roll with the changes. When we rest, we settle into an experience of consciousness that has no preference or needs. This is different to sleep, when we might be dreaming and working through a fear or desire, and it is also a far step from the activities we might do to relax, which inevitably involve some form of stimulus, and then thoughts and feelings about that stimulus. Whether your experience as rest comes as a momentary middle-distance gaze (so precious, and so very absent now we have our smartphones to fill in every gap) or a longer, deliberate process of letting go (perhaps through a yoga nidra class, or via the Enquiries in this book), you will become more aware of your invincible, essential self:

- *Find a comfortable space, preferably lying down in a way that you feel most able to settle for some time. If you prefer to sit up, then do*

- *Take a few moments to observe the physical sensations in your body, such as heat, a softening, tension, perhaps a pulsing or numbness (feeling nothing is still a sensation). Start at the top – the crown of your head – and work down to the* tips of your toes. You can go deep, such as exploring the insides of your ears, the roof of your mouth, the spaces between your ribs. Take your time, linger over the details, and only note the physical feelings (not your preferences for them, or what they might mean)

- Notice any stronger sensations that may become feelings (such as warmth in the heart, heaviness in the tummy) and emotions (sadness, delight) that might begin to emerge. Notice how your mind might draw conclusions or want to make a story out of these. See if you can simply stay with the raw feelings in the body

- Invite your thoughts to come and go just as they please. Make a pact with yourself not to judge the activity of your mind – if it's busy, then so be it; it doesn't mean you're doing anything wrong. Take a few moments now just to be with your thoughts, however they present themselves

- Notice how there is a 'you' watching these thoughts. Take a few minutes to consider this position as 'watcher' of the thoughts, as opposed to 'thinker' of the thoughts

- With your body–mind tour complete, just rest. Lie still for a few moments, allowing everything to be just as it is

- See if you can fall into that place of awareness that has been here all along – both at the beginning, as your witness taking a tour of your body, and then as you were, spending a moment watching your thoughts. There is part of you present, behind all the thoughts, sensations, feelings, images and sounds, which is stable, unchanging awareness

- Linger in this place of awareness for as long as you are able or feels right

- When you are ready, take a few deep breaths, stretch, wriggle and welcome yourself back

(It's Never) The End

If you've read this book all the way to its conclusion we can only assume you've enjoyed it, or are so restless that you didn't know what else to do with yourself. Either way, thank you. Thanks for reading us.

We'd like to end with a final missive: to remind you that we cannot tell you what life is all about, but we can be sure that it is and forever will be an unending mystery.

The universe in which you live is absolutely enormous. If you take a moment to look up at the night sky, you will know this to be true. What you can glimpse above you is vast open space, populated with stars – suns, bigger and brighter than our own, some many quadrillions of miles away.

What you can see is an infinitesimally small part of our galaxy, something so enormous and richly populated by these points of light and their solar systems, it's incomprehensible.

And this is just one of hundreds of billions of galaxies amid a universe that is ever-growing, continuing to expand, infinitely, in all directions.

Who you are on one hand is tiny and inconsequential, and on the other hand as infinite as the universe. Your deepest nature is that which contains everything, that which pervades everywhere, that which contains the absolute.

How and why all this *is* remains a mystery, but experiencing it is yours to feel into whenever you wish. The timeless, spacious nature of your deepest self knows no bound; it is unborn and undying.

We'd like to offer you this reflection to rest in: that who you are is inextricably part of the whole and undeniably endless. Who you are is all of this, and it's magnificent, without end.

What you live in and are part of is expanding without end, and what you are is part of it and expanding without end.

You never end.

The end.

ONE PLACE. MANY STORIES

Bold, innovative and
empowering publishing.

FOLLOW US ON:

@HQStories